Also by Fiona Giles

From the Verandah

Melanie

Dick for a Day

Too Far Everywhere

Chick for a Day

FRESH MILK

MILK

The Secret Life of Breasts

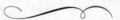

Fiona Giles

Simon & Schuster

New York   London
Toronto   Sydney   Singapore

SIMON & SCHUSTER
Rockefeller Center
1230 Avenue of the Americas
New York, NY 10020

First Simon & Schuster trade paperback edition 2003

SIMON & SCHUSTER and colophon are registered trademarks
of Simon & Schuster, Inc.

For information regarding special discounts for bulk purchases,
please contact Simon & Schuster Special Sales at 1-800-456-6798
or business@simonandschuster.com

Book design by Ellen R. Sasahara

Manufactured in the United States of America

10   9   8   7   6   5   4   3   2   1

Library of Congress Cataloging-in-Publication Data is available
ISBN 0-7432-1147-2

In memory of

Colin Alexander Hood

1956–2002

And praise will come to those whose kindness
Leaves you without debt
And bends the shape of things to come
That haven't happened yet

—NEIL FINN, "Faster Than Light"

Introduction

W henever I used to think of fresh milk, I imagined rows and rows of chilled cartons of cows' milk, neatly arranged according to their fat content or their added proteins and vitamins, and sometimes colored with chocolate, or strawberry, or caramel. When I was young, fresh milk was delivered in glass bottles to the front gate. Later it came from the corner store, or the cold food aisle of the supermarket. It listed nutritional contents on the label and the percentage these represented of the recommended daily allowance. It had a use-by date. And it had to be kept cold.

Once I began to breastfeed my children, my idea of fresh milk suddenly changed. Fresh milk is warm, and watery pale. Its packaging walks and talks, and runs, and makes love. It is absent of labeling. It has no fixed quantity, or set loading of nutrients, but ebbs and flows according to the needs of its consumers. It is flavored with garlic, or vanilla, or carrots, and sometimes all these things. It is not confined to fridges and stores, but is everywhere women are.

Western culture tends to think of women's milk only in relation to the babies they might choose to feed. We think of lactating women as immediately postpartum, still wrapped in the aura of childbirth and laden with the trappings of infancy: bassinets, strollers, blankets, diaper bags, the thousand-and-one bits and pieces that we buy when our babies arrive. It's as if we hire our new milky breasts along with all this stuff, and sign a rental contract specifying that they must be packed away and forgotten after weaning, sometime within the baby's first year. These hired lactating breasts are connected to the hospital bed, to nursing bras and nursing pads, and special diets, and sleepless nights, and hollow-eyed jealous husbands. They are medically scrutinized, gently massaged, and intensely discussed during the time they are used. Then, when the flow is stanched, they are primly returned to their lacy cage, to be admired again according to purely aesthetic considerations.

The more I researched this book, the clearer it became that breastmilk is not only a feature of maternity wards and parental bedrooms, or even those well-lit corners of shopping centers and car parks from which breastfeeding mothers have frequently been ejected. The places and conditions in which women—and children and men—experience breastfeeding are far more varied and surprising than this. But the details of how we fit breastfeeding into our lives, or decide that it doesn't fit, are not well known. And the meaning of breastfeeding—as opposed to its nutritional content—is rarely discussed outside mothers' groups and pediatricians' waiting rooms.

Of the people I spoke to, most had succeeded in fitting breastfeeding into their lives, and often in surprising ways. Early on in my research, I came across a press clipping from March 1997, about a South African mother, Kristen Grobler, who had breastfed her poodle puppy while also breastfeeding her baby. I knew about tandem-feeding, in which twins are fed simultaneously, and sometimes older and younger siblings. I'd also read about women in Papua New Guinea nursing their piglets, as these are domestic animals in that country; and women in many countries in previous centuries, including Canadian Indians and white American women, who nursed puppies, either to nourish their pets, toughen their nipples, or keep up their supply. The mythic Romulus and Remus were nursed by a wolf; and it has recently emerged that a South American orphan who was "adopted" by a pack of dogs also drank their milk. But the Johannesburg mother landed this kind of breastfeeding squarely in our contemporary suburban landscape.

Some of these events might be dismissed, in the normal course of life, as unnervingly weird. But it is curious to me why our mythology about women as producers of food from their own bodies is so incomplete. In the last twenty years we have begun to accept the full reality of women's bodies giving birth to their offspring as a cataclysmic, yet natural event—neither an illness nor a disability. Yet we still balk at the idea of these same bodies making something that all of us can drink.

The stories we do have, scattered through history, novels, and film, veer between reverential accounts drawing on the Christian myth of the selfless and virginal Madonna and Child, and smutty pop culture jokes and asides. We either have to go way back to the Renaissance, to Caravaggio's *Seven Acts of Mercy* and Peter Paul Rubens's *Venus, Mars and Cupid,* or way forward, to Liz Hurley's jugs of cream in *Austin Powers* or Jim Carrey's assault on a nursing mother in *Me, Myself, & Irene.* Pablo Picasso and Frida Kahlo are two exceptions among twentieth-century painters, who had an interest in the subject. Picasso has been quoted by the art critic Betty Churcher as saying, "Those breasts are most beautiful that give the most milk." There are scattered literary references, stories and poems by women about nursing, such as Elissa Schappell's "Here Is Comfort, Take It" in her short story collection *Use Me,* and the poems of Sharon Olds.

But these are relatively obscure, and there is very little, even in feminist nonfiction, that gazes steadily on the fully lived experience of all the people involved.

Within this fully lived realm, I learned of the vastness and diversity of people's experience with breastmilk. I heard from women who had never had children, nor even been pregnant, who produced milk during sex. Another woman, who longed to become pregnant, told me that her breasts felt heavier after she'd been cuddling her friend's baby. A grandmother who'd weaned her own children thirty years earlier said she spontaneously produced milk for her grandson, and so helped her daughter to feed him. Perfectly ordinary men confessed how they longed to drink milk from a woman's breasts, both as a sexual turn-on and as a means to deepen a friendship. Mothers who'd ceased feeding their babies told me they'd decided to keep up their supply for their husbands. Others noticed that if they squeezed their breasts, many years after weaning, droplets of milk still emerged.

I heard from mothers who topped up their family's breakfast bowls with milk from their breasts, or added it to their coffee, or the mashed potatoes. A woman whose baby died continued to pump her milk and donate it to a milk bank. A thirteen-year-old Melbourne girl was given two cups of breastmilk a day, donated by other women, to survive her allergies. A New Yorker, who wasn't breastfed as a child, told me of his curiosity about the flavor of breastmilk and offered to make it into ice cream for me if I could find a donor. A father told me how he'd comforted his daughter by letting her latch onto his breast when the mother was away. An Englishman emailed to say he'd produced milk for his baby in the 1970s and helped his wife breastfeed. I spoke to the New York–based artist Patrick Bucklew, who was once offended by a stripper in a Provincetown club squirting milk at him, but went on to produce prosthetic breasts that squirted coconut milk ten feet and incorporate them into his own performances.

Perhaps the most surprising story from a man came from a Sydney taxi driver who told his passenger—a lactation consultant—that as a child in Bosnia he had been hired out by his dad, in exchange for cigarettes, to relieve nursing mothers of their engorgement by sucking their breasts. He told the lactation consultant with some pride, "Some days I sucked tit before school, and some days after school. The ladies thought I was cute so they gave me cakes and sweets after I finished. Some days I was so full of milk and cakes I had a bellyache."

I heard from large-breasted women who had discovered they could breastfeed themselves, and one of them added this to her repertoire when masturbating. After one interview I conducted for this book, I experienced the feeling of letdown, as though my milk were coming in, even though I'd not breastfed for over a year.

I could only conclude that there is much more breastmilk in our lives, in our bodies, and in our culutral imaginary, than we realize. Through my research, it has gradually made itself known to me, almost as if it is a great lost resource of contemporary life.

In addition to listening to stories, I also sent out questionnaires, and received over two hundred replies, mostly from women but approximately 10 percent from men. Replies came from Australia, America, New Zealand, Canada, Britain, South Africa, and France. I used the questionnaires to find more stories and to get a broad, qualitative picture of the attitudes to breastfeeding in our culture. Naturally, I received many more answers from breastfeeding enthusiasts than any other kind. But within that group there exists not only an incredible breadth of wisdom and expertise on the subject, but also a startling variety of views on what is right, or wrong, or difficult, or joyful about breastfeeding today. As any expectant mom who's read up on the subject knows, there are almost as many methods for breastfeeding as there are babies, and breasts to put them on.

Fresh Milk is a selection of the stories I encountered. It is a galaxy of voices, a narrative Milky Way. Some of the stories grew out of answers to the questionnaire, others are edited from interviews, and several are based on email exchanges. Some of the monologues are based on transcripts without any significant alteration, while others are based on combined voices, and have been fictionalized. Three of the stories were written by other women—Gayle Brandeis, Belinda Luscombe, and Alison Bartlett—and adapted for this collection. Many of the names in the stories have been changed to protect the privacy of contributors and their children.

All the stories are based on the experiences, memories, and research of people who have been touched by breastfeeding, or its absence. Together they extend the boundaries of what we consider normal when it comes to human parenting. They reveal a glimpse of what lactation means to us, and how it might fit more amply into our lives. *Fresh Milk* is an oral history in the fullest sense of the word, abundant and overflowing. Enjoy!

FRESH
MILK

Mammatocumulus

⌒━━━━━⌒

The association between breastfeeding and the sky is ancient, though not well known. The term *galaxy*, or Milky Way, derives from the same term for lactation—*galactic*—as does the term *galactagogue*, which is any type of food or chemical that is thought to increase a mother's supply. In South America there exists a cow tree (*Galactodendron utile*), which produces a milky sap called galactin that can be used as a cream. There is also a geological formation, the mamelon, which resembles an outcrop of gigantic nipples and was featured in Peter Weir's 1975 film *Picnic at Hanging Rock*.

The story of the Milky Way, as it appears in Greco-Roman mythology, concerns the feeding of baby Hercules, son of Jupiter. Because Hercules' mother was mortal, Zeus put Hercules to the breast of the Goddess Juno, his wife and sister, knowing that Hercules would acquire immortality through her milk. As Hercules suckled from the sleeping Juno's breast, she woke up and pushed him away. As she did so her milk sprayed across the heavens, crystallizing into a promontory of stars. Her milk that fell on the ground produced lilies. The myth is depicted in many classical paintings, such as Tintoretto's sixteenth-century masterpiece *The Origin of the Milky Way*.

The first story is by American writer Gayle Brandeis, who tells of another, even less well-known breastly phenomenon in the skies.

⁓

My breasts hang inside my dress like soft tongues. They loll against the cotton, barely tasting the fabric. My nipples are not as responsive as they once were. Perhaps all the nursing I did—four and a half years total between the two kids—sucked the nerve endings of my nipples numb. Now it takes great cold, or my husband's great mouth, to bring them out of their soft shell.

After I swim, I am always so happy to look down and see my nipples poke hard against the Spandex of my bathing suit. It reminds me I am still alive, still sentient, still capable of involuntary excitement.

I find myself staring at women's breasts. I'm as bad as a stereotypical man, forcing myself to look into women's eyes when my gaze keeps drifting downward. The different shapes and sizes of mammary glands fascinate me no end. I wonder, "What is it like to live with those breasts? And those? And those?"

This obsession doesn't feel sexual. I think my paucity of breast tissue makes me curious about those who have more, like a girl in a bakery, happy with her small cookies, but gaping in awe at the huge cakes dripping with frosting all around her. I guess I have breasts on the brain. When I was fixated on my teeth, I stared at everyone's mouth.

I see breasts in the sky. I recently learned a mammatocumulus is a storm cloud with breast-shaped protuberances hanging from its belly. I expect to lift my face to the gathering storm and be showered with warm milk, sweet and abundant.

When my son was a baby, I squirted breastmilk into the batter of one of the pumpkin pies my sister and I baked for Thanksgiving. The breastmilk pie had a much deeper, richer color than the one with condensed cows' milk in it, but it didn't hold together quite so well.

At thirty-two my breasts are not holding together quite so well themselves. They are crone breasts, lined and tired looking. After my daughter weaned and the milk slowly receded into my body, I remember thinking my breasts looked forlorn. My left breast seems melancholy even now, hanging solemnly on my chest, its nipple still creased from the sudden deflation. When I bend forward, my breasts sag into two little sacks beneath me, empty bota bags.

Clarissa Pinkola Estes writes: "Does it feed? Does it feel? It is a good breast." I have written a book to teach women to love their own bodies, but I still need to repeat this quote to myself, over and over, again and again.

When my son nursed, his upper lip undulated like a centipede. He could stay there for hours. My daughter would take a few little sucks at a time, then look away, more interested in the world than what my body could offer.

I remember nursing my kids in the car, hanging my body over the car seat. Nursing standing up. Nursing in the bathtub. Nursing on the floor with the baby lying on my belly, craning her neck to reach my breast. Like inventive lovers, we found ourselves in all kinds of positions, anytime, anyplace.

At the Lincoln Park Zoo last August, I watched a gorilla baby nurse from his mama. Both of them lay side by side on their backs, looking up at the tall ceiling of the gorilla house. One long, dark nipple stretched from her chest to his mouth like an extension cord. Their eyes looked blissed out, glazed with the hormones and sweet comfort of lactation. I remember that floating, spacy, warm feeling so well.

I see that look, too, in the photo of an ethnic Albanian woman on the cover of an April 1999 issue of *Time*. She is nursing her baby while she walks to a refugee camp in Macedonia. Her hands clutch the blanket the baby is wrapped in, a thick white synthetic-looking throw, covered with starbursts. Her dark eyes are filled with fear and exhaustion, but I see a calmness in them too, a gauzy nursing gaze that I hope made the difficult march out of Kosovo more bearable. The magazine still sits in an organizer on my desk. I look at the woman's eyes often.

I was so angry when I saw a couple of adolescent boys ogling her in the checkout line of the grocery store. They elbowed each other and laughed and pointed to her exposed breast, soft and round, emerging from her leather jacket. There were plenty of posed, pushed-up breasts on other magazine covers that they could have drooled at, but this was a real breast before them, unguarded and true. I pulled the magazine from the rack and held it to my own breasts. I carried the picture of my fellow mother-sister with me, back to my secure home.

My great-grandmother was killed during a pogrom in Russia when she was nearing her due date. My grandfather watched as a Cossack raped her, his mother, then slit her large belly open. I wonder if her colostrum had come in yet, rising from her nipples like drops of amber, something that could preserve history.

Sometimes a thin silvery crust, like a sugar glaze, still forms over my nipples, over four years after the last weaning. I carefully pick it from my body, leaving small pink craters on the tips of my nipples. A hint of sweetness rises from beneath my nails. I put my fingers to my tongue, and my mouth fills with longing.

Quest for Bravura:
The Expensive Perils
of Shopping for a
Nursing Bra

S hopping is one of the most daunting challenges of expectant motherhood. The list seems infinite, from baby books to baths and booties, plus the furniture that ends up soon after the birth in garage sales, barely used.

It might be thought that shopping for maternity clothes should be easier; and it's more fun now that the outline of the pregnant belly has become acceptable, and the floral tent dress with Peter Pan collar is pretty much a thing of the past.

But if my own experience is anything to go by, the real lesson is that normal clothes, including men's shirts, and jackets, dresses or leggings that stretch, and the beauty of a bare belly are in most cases just as good.

Could this also be true for underwear? It's tempting to think so.

I went looking for my first nursing bra when I was about four months pregnant with my first son. I was on holiday in my hometown of Perth, so I gravitated without thinking toward the large department stores that I'd trawled as a teenager looking for foxy boob tubes and purple stretch jeans. As a small-breasted individual I'd only ever worn seamless, unlined bras, having no real need for support and no desire to look bigger. So I'd been harboring the fantasy of now graduating to something lusciously overblown, padded and underwired.

The shop assistant was horrified at the idea of using a normal underwire bra in pregnancy and for nursing. "You'll crush your milk ducts!" she cried. And I was marched across to the proper nursing bra section where, I was informed, underwire was banished. But other means of containment were clearly in full use, as we seemed to have stepped back in time to a 1950s foundation garment store.

Not that there were many to choose from, but they all looked horrifyingly prosthetic. The pink-toned beige had the flesh-colored look of a fake body part straining to blend in. These were items suffering from aesthetic shame, and desperate to vanish.

But this was a lost cause—they were too big. Their outsize dimensions were designed not just to encompass something undeniably large, but to regulate untoward fleshy bits and mold them into a strictly decorous shape. The multiple clasps on the inches-wide back strap were reminiscent of Victorian corsetry. But I was meanwhile being assured by my guide that these forbidding structures were carefully designed with safety, hygiene, and convenience in mind. Clearly no consideration for the exquisite sensibilities of recently nubile breasts was permitted.

My matronly helper, who herself seemed to have stepped out of a Doris Day movie, proceeded to explain how the width of the straps would support even the most engorged breast. These worked together with the bracelike back strap and a strip of fabric underneath each cup, which was said to perform the same function as underwire, but without risking the aforementioned crushing tendencies.

I was feeling somewhat crushed myself at this point, and had begun to mutter something about not really knowing how big my breasts would become when I reached full term, and perhaps I should be on my way. But my guide was not to be put off so easily, and firmly told me that I should buy something as soon as possible, and most definitely before giving birth, because my pregnant breasts needed proper support right now. I should also buy a second bra two cup sizes larger, she advised, going from my new size C to a DD, which would be suitable once my milk came in.

Blinded by science, or perhaps just by disappointment, I allowed her to usher me into a dressing room with several beige undergarments to try on. She stayed, as is the tradition with this generation of bra experts, so she could fit me properly, tilt me forward, and ease those parts that fell sideways into their proper flight path. I was trapped, in more ways than one.

She then demonstrated the various techniques used for unfastening each cup, to allow for feeding. One involved press studs at the center, between the breasts. Another had tricky plastic clips at the top, against each shoulder strap. These were clearly designed to elevate the blood pressure through frustration, as to well as break fingernails and fray tempers to shreds. And that was in a tranquil dressing room, without a screaming baby to help things along. (I've since learned these devices are called "flick and flip" clips, which seems apt considering their swift effect on mental health.)

Both bras were equally hideous to look at, but it was my fate to choose one, so I left with the plainest, and easiest to manage. I was at least confident in the ongoing well-being of my recently imperiled milk ducts.

But I didn't give up my search for something with style, especially after giving birth. I swiftly realized I had no intention of hiding my breastfeeding from the world, or denying my hungry baby, for as stupid a reason as sartorial blight. Shopping for an attractive nursing bra reminded me of looking for a sun hat in the 1980s, when the only women's hats on the market were designed for a day at the races, and I ended up having to buy a man's Panama at great expense since I didn't want to look like the Queen Mother. The point is, there were just one or two glimmers of change on the shopper's horizon—lace and bright colors, and even animal prints, slowly making their way into the specialty maternity-wear stores. Like a Panama hat, they were expensive, but they had the look of something that could be worn with pleasure, and that was worth paying for, especially after walking miles to find them.

When I finally chanced upon a black cotton lace bra, that was both soft and stretchy, and—for the record—underwired, I was at last satisfied. It was not flamboyant. It just fell within the spectrum of pretty and normal. It was comfortable and gracefully contoured. The choice of colors was limited, but at least one of them was black.

Since then, specialty maternity-bra makers have continued to enliven the shelves, and retail websites, with fabrics that celebrate the nursing breast and refuse to medicalize it. The popularity of animal prints, especially, in the late 1990s tolled a timely, atavistic death knell for the clinical nursing bra of old. And the new generation allowed for underwire, which when properly fitted poses no harm. Their only drawback, as with all nursing bras, is the inflated prices.

But then I went one better. My sister-in-law had a baby and showed me the way. As a frequent buyer of Jean Paul Gaultier and Akira Isagawa, it was obvious that no bandage-colored nylon-elastane mix was ever destined to frame her tawny cleavage. And no tacky press studs or enraging plastic clips either. Instead, she purchased several pairs of lacy, low-cut Yves Saint Laurent underwire bras, in rich hues of emerald and ruby. She had figured out that the cut was low enough and the lace flexible enough for her simply to stretch it aside while feeding. She also knew well that subtle dishevelment goes a long way, and a single bra strap draped across a bicep is sexy if executed with deliberation. If the bras wore out faster, then that was a risk she was prepared to take.

But they didn't. And like all good sisters-in-law, she passed them on to me when her daughter weaned at two years and I became pregnant for a second, much wiser time.

Letdown

S ometimes, even with the best will in the world, an ample milk supply, and aid from highly qualified lactation consultants, breastfeeding just doesn't work. The hoped-for marriage of baby to breast steadfastly refuses to be arranged by the well-meaning, adequately resourced, and hyperinformed mama.

This was the experience of journalist Belinda Luscombe when she attempted to breastfeed her son in 1997. The story she writes here is about her eventual triumph, when everything falls into place after the birth of her daughter, three years later. But the pain and disappointment from her first attempt is something she hasn't forgotten, and it turns out that even when she successfully feeds, pain—and a certain amount of comic alienation—is still an issue.

Nor is Belinda's case rare. Many of the women who responded to my questionnaire pointed out the need for realistic warnings about the potential for both pain and failure, and the need for more accessible and better informed help. Many women commented on the contradictory advice they were given, and the lack of adequately trained health professionals. One woman was appalled by the widespread ignorance, and wrote, "The amount of cobblers I got told by people who knew nothing, but thought a string of letters after their name meant they were qualified to give advice!"

Other women who faced difficulties were taken aback by their own clumsiness—something they'd not been prepared for. Writes one: "I think I was shocked at how difficult breast-feeding was. I expected it to be automatic. The process of learning to feed reminded me of learning to catch and throw a ball—both of which I was fairly hopeless at as a child. I felt humiliated at times by the nurses in the hospital. Not because they were trying to humiliate me, just because I'm not used to failing at things repeatedly. And I could see that they were getting a bit exasperated with me by the end."

A midwife who herself suffered from a cracked nipple, and had previously observed the torment of other mothers struggling to get it right, commented on the importance of adequate guidance. She writes, "I truly believe breastfeeding is certainly very much a cognitive process rather than just being at chest level!"

If all else fails, ideally a mother would have access to breastmilk from other sources, such as milk banks (which are reemerging in America, and will soon be established in Australia) or wet nurses—or maybe one day, screened and sterilized breastmilk from the corner store. But since these alternatives are unlikely to become available anytime soon, it would be just as well to downplay the virtuous rhetoric and point out instead that there are a few compensations when using formula. Longer sleeps, sharing the feeds between family members, and saving money on the exorbitant cost of nursing bras spring to mind. One older respondent pointed out to me, too, that breastfeeding was not everything, in her experience, and doesn't guarantee a perfect bill of health. She told me that although her mother breastfed her, she then failed to send her to school with any lunch, so that by the time she was a teenager all her teeth had fallen out. (I guess this mother wasn't handy with a toothbrush either!)

Whatever decision the mother ultimately makes, we need to acknowledge that breastfeeding, though a function of the body, is deeply embedded in cultural practice. It is also dependent on the right support for the entire mothering enterprise—not just for breastfeeding. As one mother is quoted saying in *The Hip Mama Survival Guide* by Ariel Gore, "Natural, my butt. We are not born with any innate ability to nurse. Don't ask me how the first people ever figured it out." Perhaps the same could be said for parenting overall.

❦

The other day I thought I was having a heart attack. But nope, it turns out I was just breastfeeding again. The gripping pain in my chest was what the lactation consultants call letdown. Letdown occurs when the milk glands spring into life and release their milk. Let down is also how you feel when you realize that breastfeeding is not as easy as it looks in those Madonna and Child paintings. To me, breastfeeding is beatific in the same way that crucifixion is holy.

There seems to be some kind of conspiracy about this, with movies, TV shows, and the aforementioned medieval paintings depicting mothers effortlessly plonking their newborn babes on their breasts as if it were as simple as riding a bike. It *is* as simple as riding a bike; remember how many times you fell off? In fact, for many women, breastfeeding is a pain in the, well, lots of places. It isn't intuitive, it isn't simple, and it's learned the same way most things are, by doing it less wrong each time. Nobody who has read the research will contest that breastfeeding is better for Junior than the options. Even the formula-makers put this on their packaging. But that doesn't make it easy.

The breastfeeding books, of which I have burned more than many people have bought, say, often in all capital letters, BREAST-FEEDING SHOULD NOT HURT. Well, apparently my breasts can't read. After three weeks of trying to nurse my now three-year-old son, during which time he gained absolutely no weight and developed a permanent sweat ring where I held his little head in a viselike grip while trying not to scream, I weaned him. I was furious—at the books, at the La Leche League, but most of all at my breasts. I wanted to tattoo "For Decorative Purposes Only; Not to Be Given to Small Children" on them.

When I had another child, I decided to try to assuage my guilt in a more productive way. I signed up for a breastfeeding class. I joined a breastfeeding support group. I rented a pump, bought nipple shells, special La Leche League–approved lanolin, three special Canadian Bravado nursing bras, and a doughnut-shaped nursing pillow called "My Brest Friend" (bad puns are to maternity goods what khaki is to the Gap). My mother crossed an ocean and a continent to cook and clean so I could focus on nursing. A lovely lactation consultant called Anastasia gave me her home number. I began to watch other women nurse and envy their nipples. Breasts occupied my every waking thought. It was like being a guy.

And still it was torture; eight to ten excruciating daily milk-sodden wrestling matches between my tiny child and my uncooperative, sore, increasingly chafed bazungas. It's a wicked cycle. The last thing you want is anyone touching your breasts; the first thing you want is to feed your child. The more you feed, the better the whole thing works. It's just hard to persuade yourself of this as you get your smarting boobs out again for another round of ritual torture.

To make matters worse, breastfeeding is the seventh circle of advice hell. Everybody has something to tell you, much of it contradictory. When I contracted mastitis, one lactation consultant told me to point my child's nose to where the blockage was; another told me to point her chin toward the blockage. One mother said to make sure I completely emptied my breasts; another said that breasts are never truly empty. A nurse said to let the baby feed as long as she wanted; a pediatrician said to nurse for no longer than twenty minutes at a time. Even the sane books have some ridiculous suggestions. *The Complete Guide to Breastfeeding,* one of the better primers, proposes that you repeat this mantra to yourself: "I am a bounteous supplier of milk for my baby." Who even uses the word *bounteous?*

The things that, unlike mantras, actually seemed to help were, if possible, even more humiliating. Wearing cool cabbage leaves against my breasts seemed to alleviate discomfort, but if I fed in public, I first had to remove wilted, slightly cooked cabbage leaves, and afterward replace them with fresh ones. To add to the mortification, I began to notice just how malodorous half-cooked cabbage is.

Why the silence about the difficulty of breastfeeding? Why all the propaganda instead of frank talk? Probably because the pendulum has swung as far as it can away from formula. Many of the women now having babies were formula-fed as infants; our mothers were advised it was somehow barbaric to nurse, that in civilized societies, children were fed this yummy gunk from cans. (An indication of how smart formula-makers think mothers are comes from the warning label on each can of powdered formula: Add water before feeding.) This trend, and I say this with a certain smugness, as I was breastfed, was regrettable and a correction was necessary. But can we not all agree that the research on breastfeeding now clearly suggests it's a worthwhile thing to do without trying to make out that it's as easy as breathing?

If the almost weekly results of studies are to be believed, breastfeeding will make your child smarter, healthier, and probably even better-looking. Fine. Let's do it. But did Karenna Gore Schiff really have to rub in how easy she found it by suggesting a march on Washington of breastfeeding moms? Does she have any idea what kind of a balancing act that would be for me, baby, the My Brest Friend, the nursing pads, and my extra-large bottle of water?

As it turns out, I am still breastfeeding my daughter, who is now thirteen months old. After the 1,539th feed (but who's counting?), it has stopped being so painful. I'm reluctant to give up, either because it took so much effort to get this far, or because I enjoy it. Or maybe it's just because as a working mother of two, I need any excuse to sit down. I would also advise anyone to breastfeed, if they could. But I want to issue a warning to all you well-meaning types who are planning breastfeeding books: If you say that letdown may be accompanied by a "tingling sensation," I will come after you with a colonoscope. And my proctologist warns me that could be "uncomfortable."

One Single Change

What single change to the world would have made breastfeeding easier for you?*

Men having breasts.

Comfy chairs when out and about.

Better-educated doctors.

More acceptance of breastfeeding in public.

Breast pads that work and don't look as though I have two small dinner plates attached to my chest.

Having everyone do it so I wouldn't have to discuss it constantly.

More comfortable bras.

More acceptance of breastfeeding in public.

Regular visits from a lactation consultant.

Allowing for "forbidden" practices, like test-weighing and nipple shields, to be tried if other things fail.

Being able to feed my baby at work.

More acceptance of breastfeeding in public.

Advice and help from people who actually knew what the hell they were talking about.

More images of breasts as a food source rather than a sex thing.

Better prenatal education.

* Answers to this and following questions in the book were selected from replies to the questionnaire.

More acceptance of breastfeeding in public.

Better-designed baby changing rooms, better feeding facilities, and armchairs in ladies' rooms specifically for breastfeeding.

To share the duty of breastfeeding with someone else, and not have to do it at night.

Knowing that all types of mothers breastfeed, not just the ones that everyone thinks are the "good mommies."

More acceptance of breastfeeding in public.

For cross-species feeding to be seen as abnormal.

More milk banks, and powdered human milk.

Understanding the benefits of extended breastfeeding for both mother and child.

More acceptance of breastfeeding in public.

No thrush.

More interaction with other nursing mothers in the early stages.

If my husband could have done some of it.

More acceptance of breastfeeding in public.

Being less tired.

Fewer carcinogens in our diets and cities and households to get stored up in my breasts in order to be passed on to my baby!

Getting help for my cracked nipples earlier.

That we all had the option to walk around topless.

More acceptance of breastfeeding in public.

Situations Vacant

On the last page of Valerie Fildes's *Wet Nursing: A History from Antiquity to the Present,* published in 1988, she mentions a rare case of a young mother in Claremont, Western Australia, who advertised in her local paper for a wet nurse. Virtually unheard-of today, wet-nursing was commonplace among the middle classes of Europe and England in the eighteenth and nineteenth centuries. While it saved many babies' lives when mothers had died or were unable to produce milk, it was also a cause of suffering and death among the children of mothers whose only source of income was to breastfeed the children of their more affluent employers. It was also popular in the aristocratic classes of countries where large families were a priority. If a mother weaned early by passing her children on to a wet nurse, she could then fall pregnant again much sooner.

Since there were no safe alternatives to breastmilk, wet-nursing remained popular until the end of the nineteenth century, when pasteurization of cows' milk meant that babies fed by artificial means would be less likely to die from infection. It continued well into the 1940s, according to Fildes, with many young women turning to wet-nursing, often through hospital-based schemes, to supplement their income. In America, directories of wet nurses were set up in Boston, New York, and Philadelphia. This meant that a certain degree of regulation was possible, both for the quality of the wet nurse and the wages she could receive. Photos from the 1920s, now held at the Smithsonian, show groups of wet nurses in a Chicago hospital, attired in sterile masks and gowns, expressing milk to be stored for premature and sick infants. It is interesting that many doctors from this era continued to promote regulated wet-nursing as an alternative to what they saw as inferior cows' milk–based substitutes. But formula became the increasingly popular option for mothers in difficulty. And the medical profession began to promote formula as superior, exploiting a post-Victorian, middle-class squeamishness that saw breastfeeding as unrefined, even beastly. At the same time, women's professional choices began to improve, particularly after they had proved themselves able workers during the two world wars, so that wet-nursing as a means of earning an income became less important.

By the 1980s, when the Western Australian mother, Beth Taylor, considered advertising for someone to feed her daughter on the afternoons when she studied, the practice of wet-nursing was so rare that the term was unknown to her. It was her mother who pointed out that it was once a profession, and had a name.

Wet-nursing, or at least cross-nursing, in which close friends or relatives nurse each other's babies on a casual basis, is perhaps more common than we realize. The official policy of the La Leche League, the principal breastfeeding advocacy and support group in America, is to discourage the practice, due to a fear of infections that might be passed on to the baby through breastmilk by women who unknowingly suffer from HIV-AIDS, or hepatitis C. And a substitute nursing mother might not be as vigilant about being free of nicotine or other drugs and alcohol. But as Beth Taylor notes in her story, groups of women who are well known to each other and frequently baby-sit each other's children sometimes agree to share their milk.

The majority of women who answered my questionnaire stated that they would be willing to nurse someone else's child if a mother was in need and asked them. It was a rare respondent who said she would find this repugnant, or unnatural. And several women confessed to cross-nursing, with consent, as an occasional backup between friends or sisters while baby-sitting.

As Valerie Fildes writes: "It is ironic that some of the groups promoting breastfeeding disapprove of cross nursing, because of the risk of infection and possible interference with the mother-child bonding process: two of the main reasons why wet nursing has been condemned [by some] since antiquity. However, it is interesting to find that mothers who do nurse babies other than their own do not report distaste, or other negative feelings, towards the practice. Most find it enjoyable and 'natural'; some felt closer to these babies than before they suckled them, and continued to feel closer to them than to children whom they had not breastfed."

WET Nurse/nursing mother. Few hours
per week. 3 month baby. Mother studies.
Reciprocation or remuneration 555 3296.

—*Claremont Nedlands Post,* March 3, 1987

M y daughter Leia was three months old when I advertised in
the local paper for a wet nurse. One of the journalists saw
my ad and my story ended up on the front page.

When Leia was born I was twenty-six. I was working to set up
my own practice in Occupational Therapy, and I had enrolled in a
graduate diploma in health sciences at Curtin University. Leia
wouldn't take the bottle, and I didn't like expressing. My husband
was prepared to bring her to me when I was studying, but at the last
minute the university changed the course hours, and he couldn't
do it.

Probably because of the newspaper article, I got four applica-
tions. None of the women I spoke to wanted to be paid. They felt it
was part of us all being women together.

I interviewed two women on the phone. One was too far away. I
can't remember why I decided the other woman wouldn't have
worked out.

The other two women I went to see. One was married with four
children, and the youngest two she was still feeding were twins. She

was amazing—one of those women who do so many things at once, all of them wonderfully. But she lived in the other direction from the university.

I chose Susan, a single mom in her early twenties. Her twelve-month-old daughter was still nursing, but only twice a day. The main thing I remember about Susan is that she was adopted. That was the big thing in her life. She had only just met her mother when she was pregnant, and the meeting had gone pretty well. She lived in Gray-lands, which was on the way to the university from my home in Fre-mantle.

We had a lovely friendship. I spent a lot of time at her place, and we'd have long talks. We always spent time together while Leia was there, not only for her sake, but because I really liked Susan's com-pany. But when my course stopped we didn't keep in touch for very long. We did see each other a couple of times, but then we lost contact.

I never looked after her baby when she went out. I didn't nurse her, as she was down to only morning and nighttime feeds. But Susan said that her daughter did become more interested in breastfeeding again when she saw her feeding Leia.

My mother had breastfed me for six months when I was born in 1956, in Malaya. My father had been seconded to the British Army, and Mom was surrounded by upper-class English women who wouldn't breastfeed. They thought it was dirty. When she had my younger brother in 1959 we were living in Perth and she donated her extra milk to the Bethesda Hospital. She didn't have any difficulty with the idea of me using a wet nurse, although she was a little taken aback, I think. But she was also surprised that she hadn't thought of it as an option.

The newspaper article certainly sparked lots of conversations—between my friends and between my mother and her friends. People I hadn't heard from in years suddenly got in touch. Everyone was interested.

There were several letters to the paper in the following weeks about my ad. Many of them were worried about disease. And my hairdresser was horrified, but only because I'd allowed myself to be photographed before I'd had my hair cut! In the photo Jay, Leia's older brother, is smiling, as he smiled at everyone. But Leia had this look. She was easygoing, but she just wasn't a smiling baby. She scrutinized her world very carefully.

I've never known a child to object to being fed by another woman. We used to do it regularly in Darwin, where I lived when Jay was born. That's why it seemed such a normal thing for me. There was a group of six or seven of us who looked after each other's babies, and if a child needed feeding, then whoever was there would feed it. I remember when Jay was tiny, I fed a friend's six-month-old baby, and thought, "Gee, their sucking power gets much stronger!"

In Darwin in the early eighties AIDS wasn't an issue. There were no communicable diseases that concerned us then. Later on in Perth I wasn't concerned about AIDS as it wasn't common among women at that time. And it's not the way I think of people. I relate to things and make decisions on the basis of trust.

In Darwin I didn't even know the term *wet nurse*. We didn't call it by any name. We just fed one another's children, like we'd feed an older child a banana if it was hungry. We didn't make anything of it. It was only when I was talking with my mother about finding someone to feed Leia that I learned the term.

Being part of that group in Darwin, it felt like there was more than one mother for any child in the community. To be able to feed another woman's child made me feel that between us all, there was a tribe there somewhere. I felt like a part of that tribe, rather than being bonded to any one baby I'd nursed. We were just part of a community, held in a container of all of us.

The Other Woman

~

The following story is set in New Zealand in the mid-1990s, and was covered in the press in many countries. Here the mother, Pam Sutton, tells the story in her own words about the time her baby was breastfed by another woman without her knowledge or consent.

At the time Pam's story was reported in the media, some women who had not had children found it difficult to understand her anger toward the stranger who breastfed her daughter. But from the answers I received to my questionnaire, I learned that while the majority of women would agree to nurse another woman's child under certain conditions, or have their own child nursed by another, all stressed the need for consent in cross-nursing relationships.

Although intrusions on intimacy were sometimes cited, or a sense that the mother's milk would be best tailored to the needs of her own child, often the reasons were health-related. Nevertheless, several women answering the questionnaire confessed to feeding a friend's baby but not telling. As one wrote: "I once nursed a friend's baby while I was baby-sitting him. I never told my friend about it; I was worried about what she would think. Her baby was completely miserable, and I was at the end of my rope, so I finally decided to put him to my breast. It was funny—he obviously wasn't used to the shape of my nipple, and it was a bit awkward, but it did calm him down."

An extremely touching story came from a woman whose first baby was put out to adoption at two and a half weeks, a decision she bitterly regretted. She wrote: "When I lost my first child, I breastfed my sister's child without asking her. I longed to breastfeed again, any child."

In one reply, a woman writes, "I would nurse another person's baby, absolutely. I remember now that I tried to as a child when I baby-sat once!" Perhaps as breastfeeding becomes more commonplace again, this is something we will have to educate our children, and our baby-sitters, about.

Some women even expressed a willingness to feed a baby of another species, if it were in need. Wrote one: "I would have been happy to nurse a baby of any species." While some specified they would nurse only a baby gorilla or monkey, because it would feel close to a human baby, others confessed to having fed their pets. An adventurous lactation consultant wrote: "I have also nursed a baby puppy, who was being fed by a mother cat at the time. I wanted to feel what it was like. It felt like tugging, and almost tickled. I was amazed he continued to suck from my breast even though there was no milk, that I could see anyway."

Some women worried about sharp teeth. As performance artist Diane Torr pointed out, having noted that her own baby was "more like a creature that burrows underground than a person": "I would definitely be game to try it. It depends on whether it was a baby tiger or a baby pig!" Another woman wrote that she wouldn't nurse an animal, but stated: "I have expressed and kept a baby rabbit alive on my milk until he was old enough to release." Another woman remembered a similar case, writing: "A friend of mine gave all her frozen expressed milk to her dogs when she had finished feeding her baby, rather than pour it down the sink."

Although these incidents were exploratory or health-related, cross-nursing can also be a religious act. Marilyn Yalom writes in *A History of the Breast* that Veronica Giuliana, a medieval nun, slept with a young lamb and "nursed it in memory of the lamb of God. For this extreme act of piety she was beatified in the fifteenth century by Pope Pius II."

In most cases of cross-nursing reported in the questionnaires, it was merely a practical arrangement where sisters or friends had agreed in advance that if their baby was in need and the mother was absent, they would take over. Some said it felt different, or "a bit strange," while for others it was an unexpected chance to deepen a relationship with a niece or nephew.

In Muslim culture, this deepening of intimacy is officially recognized in the Koran, which states that any breastfed child immediately becomes related to its nurse, and is subsequently forbidden from marrying into her family.

Our own culture makes no such official recognition of kinship ties, but the connection is perhaps still there, at an informal level. As one man wrote, in his reply to the questionnaire for fathers, "I would encourage the feeding of other people's children if it was necessary. I often speak of Naomi, from the Old Testament, who relactated to feed her grandchild while Ruth, the mother, went to war after her husband was killed."

Like Ruth, populations at war, in exile, or needing to travel long distances to work are more likely to avail themselves of cross-feeding arrangements. As one Mexican mother told her breastfeeding counselor in Texas, her own mother had taken over the breastfeeding of her eldest child after she'd been forced to migrate alone to America to find work.

When enacted safely and with consent, cross-feeding can provide a strong link between generations, relatives, and friends. Enacted irresponsibly, as the following story suggests, it can become yet another symptom of a social fragmentation that can cruelly affect mothers, who are, on the whole, expected to raise their children alone.

A great deal of information is in the literature with regard to disease transmission via breastfeeding/human milk, and care must be taken to ensure safety.

—Mary E. Tagge, "Wet Nursing 2001"

Natasha, my second child, was about eight months old when she went with me to a Parent Center conference, an occasion where breastfeeding would be discussed. I was a delegate for our region, Mana, in the lower North Island of New Zealand. The conference was held on campus at a boy's boarding school, so those of us with babies and youngsters were put up in dormitories. We had the option of having our children with us, attending all the workshops, but I thought that it was good to have a bit of a break, so I put Natasha in the day-care center that was on-site.

The day-care center people knew everyone's timetable, and they had runners who would come and get us if our babies were in need. If it was in the middle of a business session they'd put up an overhead, such as, "Baby Michael Smith needs his mommy," that sort of thing.

I'd go and see Natasha as often as I could, and she was fine. The people looking after her commented that she was the happiest baby there, and that they'd never heard her cry.

The first night, they came and got me from a meeting for her evening feed. The next night we were at the annual presentation of certificates, and I was receiving an award for leadership. The babies that night were being looked after by a baby-sitting firm. Natasha had gone down a bit earlier than usual, and I was anticipating that she'd need a feed round about 9:00 or 9:30 P.M. Nine o'clock came, and I was getting a bit edgy, sitting at my table with my friends, and I said, "Maybe I should go back. I should see if she's all right."

We were a hundred yards away in the hall. And my friends said, "Pam, she'll be fine, just enjoy yourself. They'll come and get you if she needs you. She's probably just having one of those extra sleeps."

And I'm going, "Yeah, yeah, I'm probably being silly about it."

About eleven o'clock I left, as that was our curfew time for the babies. There were half a dozen women there, picking their babies up. Natasha was sitting in the arms of one of the mothers, and quite happy. So I said, "Hallo, darling, what are you doing up? You all right?"

The other woman said, "She is now."

I looked at her a bit funny, and she said, "I fed her."

I was gobsmacked. I just reached out and took Natasha from this woman. It took me a full minute just to register what had happened. This woman had breastfed my baby. I could tell from the way she said it that it wasn't like she gave her formula, or a drink of water, or anything like that.

I get upset quite easily, and I can blow, but in this situation I remained completely calm. I thought, If I start reacting, I could say and do things that I may regret, and I have to look at this rationally. I wanted to be in control of everything that was going on, so that I would remember who said what. And I didn't want to get into a big hissy fit at eleven o'clock at night.

Okay, she breastfed my baby without my consent. The other ramifications were Parent Center policy. I was thinking of social issues. The health aspect of it. Allergies run in the family, so I'm conscious of what I eat. I don't drink when I'm breastfeeding, yet I'd seen this woman drinking wine the night before. I didn't know whether she was drinking the night she breastfed my baby.

And isn't consent important? If we condone this action, that means we've given up our rights as parents, and anyone can come in and say what this child needs and give it to them.

I choose to feed my baby because my milk is best for my baby, and it's an intimate, dynamic relationship that I have no wish to share with anyone else. If I couldn't feed her, then I'd possibly choose someone to do it, and it would be consensual.

So I was very careful about what I said. I had to find out what the facts were. It's my journalist's instinct.

The baby-sitter said she felt overthrown. She said that although Natasha was quite happy, three women who had just arrived had said they'd feed her, and that I wouldn't mind. So she thought this must have been common among the Parent Center clientele.

The three women claimed Natasha was screaming hysterically. But considering that my closest friends had never heard Natasha cry, let alone scream, this is hard to believe. Even if she were screaming her lungs out, it was immaterial. The fact remains, I had paid for a service that I didn't get. The baby-sitters didn't come and get me, and they didn't use their cell phone to contact me. The mother who breastfed Natasha maintained she was doing me a favor. Ha! If she wanted to help, she could have come and got me. Bottom line.

I found out afterward that this woman and her friends have an agreement among themselves where they cross-nurse. Fine! No problem! As long as the person you choose is healthy and observes the things you think are important, I don't see a problem with that, if you have an agreement.

I guess I could have just turned around and let it be. However, I thought, No, this is something that needs to be brought to the other delegates' attention. If there's one thing the Parent Center is about, it's making informed choices.

That night I sought out the woman, and sat down and said, "So, you fed her. Why?"

She said, "Because she needed it."

My friends cannot believe how controlled I was. And I must admit, it did surprise me. But I just kept thinking of the bigger picture. Yes, I was involved in this, but everyone else was involved as well. It started to be a bit of a crusade.

The first person I spoke to was the newly elected national president of the Parent Center. She'd been sworn in the day before, and I said, "Here's a curly one for you!" She could immediately see the implications for everyone and everything.

When I spoke to my husband, Adrian, he was madder than I was. He said, "Right, we're going to ask her to have blood tests."

We composed a letter saying that I wanted to view results of blood tests. I spoke to my doctor, and he said the risks were remote but yes, there was a chance that diseases could be passed on to my daughter through this woman's milk. He gave me a list of what these were, and I sent the letter by registered mail. I gave her a couple of weeks to respond. At the same time I wrote a letter to the baby-sitting firm because I felt they had failed to provide an adequate baby-sitting service, and that they were culpable to some degree. A month later I'd received nothing back from anyone.

I rang the police to see what I could do, and asked about laying an assault charge. That was suggested to me by someone, and I quite liked the sound of that. Because it was an unwanted action. I certainly felt violated, heaven knows! And Natasha was violated.

The thing was, a stranger put her nipple in my baby's mouth. The fact that my baby was eight months old, does that make it all right? If she was two years old, does that make it all right? What if my baby was four years old?

It's like coming home and finding your partner in bed with another woman and being told, "Oh, you weren't here and he needed it." Hallo! Get the fuck out of here!

With Natasha it was worse, because she wasn't given a choice.

Breastfeeding is not sexual. It's sensual. But it's personal and it's intimate. I don't want to share my partner. I sure as hell don't want to share breastfeeding my children.

I also approached a lawyer, and he told me it was not a sure win, but it was definitely a goer. However, the money was a barrier. Plus the ongoing emotional trauma that would come from it. And really, at the end of the day, what did I want from that? What was my outcome going to be?

I was getting more and more upset, more and more irate about how everyone was fobbing me off. The message came through our national president that the other woman said that if Adrian and I had a problem with Natasha's health being compromised, then we should get Natasha tested, because it was nothing to do with her.

So I thought, Right, if she wants to play hardball, that's fine. And that's when I realized, being a journalist, this is a public issue. There's a need to raise awareness. Even if only so that people can talk about it in their little coffee groups and come to their own conclusions.

The story broke on Monday morning of the Labor Day weekend. There can't have been much news around because it made the front page. It wasn't the lead, because there was a double shooting, with the headline "Sex Club Killing." Ours was "Stranger Breastfeeds Baby Without Consent."

My first telephone call in the morning was from one of the TV channels. And while I was setting up an interview, one of the other channels rang, so I was on two channels live that night.

Tuesday morning I got a call from National Radio, they wanted to make it that day's topic for talk-back. I said no at first, but they insisted, and I agreed. But I made the mistake of doing a taped interview instead of going on-air. I came home at midday, and my answering machine was full of messages from friends as well as strangers.

I turned on the radio just in time to hear all these arrogant, ignorant people who hadn't heard the whole story, just sound bites, and made up their own minds that I was an unfit mother who had abandoned her child. What the hell was I doing enjoying myself anyway? You're not allowed to leave your baby with anyone else!

At the same time, I had people leaving messages on my phone saying, "Good for you. Your baby was sexually assaulted. I feel so sorry for you." Which is not what I meant either.

I was getting depressed. I went to my girlfriend Megan's place. She was there when my first daughter was born. She's a childbirth and parent educator, and was still being my key supporter. Just as I arrived, her neighbor put her head over the fence and said, "I heard about that woman whose baby was breastfed, and she sounds like a bit of a nutcase."

Megan stood there looking at me, expecting me to give this person an earful. But I thought, No, Megan has to live next door to this woman, so I just let it go.

Adrian was hassled at work. He had to talk to people, defend our actions, particularly as it's a generational thing. When there was milk banking, especially for preemies, of course it was fine. My mother had enough milk for half the ward. So older people didn't get it.

"When my wife was in the home . . ." The minute you hear those words you know they're talking 1960s, 1970s, and Adrian would say, "They used to, but then they stopped doing that when they realized the dangers of transmitting disease." And then Adrian would say, "And what about consent?"

So everyone missed the issues I was trying to push. The thing was, they weren't discussing the issues, they were discussing me. They were getting personal. I was dinner party talk from Kaikoura to Bluff.

I never turned around and said this other woman was a raving loony. I don't believe she is. I just wanted her to realize the ramifications of her actions and accept the consequences. I wanted her to understand that what she did was wrong. She finally sent a letter with her blood test results, after the media got involved. Thankfully they were negative.

The baby-sitting service also sent a letter saying, "We very much regret the situation. . . ." That's not an apology. They did nothing.

There was press coverage of similar cases. People wrote letters to the editor, the women's magazines did vox pop interviews, there was a letter about a nanny who had fed her employer's baby without consent, a direct *The Hand That Rocks the Cradle* story where the mother was considering laying charges.

It all became too much. I was falling apart. I had to keep me together. And I didn't want to put my family through any more. For two weeks I didn't leave the house. I cut my hair so I wouldn't be recognized. I carried checks in my wallet for days because I couldn't face going to the bank. This is not a big town, and I was known as a journalist. Even now I can feel the tears if I put myself back into those days of waking up and thinking, "Oh God, we're still in the middle of this."

I had visions of gangs of giant lactating women roving the parks, towering over the buildings, trampling down the trees, dangling their huge breasts over the prams, drooling away, and leaking milk everywhere. Lock up your children! The Mammaries are coming! I had to amuse myself some way. If I didn't make myself laugh, I'd sink deeper, and cry.

Then there was more press in March when a magazine article came out based on an interview I'd done in November. Another magazine article in Australia came out in June. It got into the London *Daily Telegraph,* and a friend called asking, "Was that you?"

I couldn't believe something way down under had traveled so far, and he read about it! Then a girlfriend who was in the States said it was over there. It was all over the Internet. I've heard of fifteen minutes of fame, but this seemed out of proportion.

The whole thing made me feel that I wasn't there when my baby needed me. I wasn't physically right next to her, for whatever reason, when I should have been. I don't believe that she was screaming hysterically, but even if she was, whatever happened to a drink of water? She was eight months old. I had started her on solids about three weeks before the conference because I wanted her to be able to have something if I was away for a while. I wouldn't have started her on solids otherwise. They could have found mashed banana. They could have given her one of those baby rusk things, they could have given her boiled water. She drank from a cup!

My milk had coursed through my child and given her life and it was all me. It was all my own work. Adrian and I had created out of love this beautiful human being, and I had sustained her and nurtured her. Breastmilk changes its composition according to the needs of the baby, and there was nothing on the earth that was as good for Natasha as my milk.

If she'd been given a bottle of formula, I'd have been pissed off. But not as much, maybe. I'm not antiformula. I'm probreast. But it was the sense of consent being ignored. Not so much the personal violation, but the consent absolutely. And the failure to follow directions. When I leave my children with a baby-sitter I shouldn't have to say, "Oh, and please don't let anyone breastfeed my child." My trust was betrayed by this woman and by the baby-sitters who wouldn't reassure my baby that I would be there for her, and then come and get me.

We are the product of our experiences, and everything's in there, whether we like it or not. If we catalog something one way, all we have to do is push a button and it's there in a different guise. I thought I had dealt with it. I thought I had rationalized it as much as I could. But it's been four years now, and not a day goes by when I don't see a woman with a young child and I'm reminded of this time.

I've been in situations where there are babies crying and I might be looking after them. But I do other things to distract them, and I always say, "Mommy will be here soon."

Lilith's Sad Friend

The following story is a simply told fantasy by an anonymous emailer who replied to my questionnaire. After I transcribed it, I was told by a midwife, who also was still breastfeeding her third child, that she had recently breastfed a close male friend who was grieving. They were standing in a stairway, she said. It was dark and private. Her friend started to cry and laid his head on her breast. Without thinking, she "opened her shirt," and he suckled. They were old friends, and it wasn't sexual. She was merely responding to his unhappiness, and they were both comforted by it.

While I hope this book will help to reframe breastfeeding so it is no longer confined by its Madonna and Child image, at the same time it is important to acknowledge that this tradition is still rich and valid. For many women, breastfeeding is an undeniably spiritual experience, and one that will bring them closer to their children than at any other time, as well as to a deeper understanding of themselves.

Early Christian literature and art is full of examples that show Mary conferring salvation through her breastmilk, such as in the fifteenth-century Flemish painting *The Lactation of Saint Bernard*. Here the baby Jesus is removed from Mary's breast so that milk sprays into the adult Saint Bernard's waiting mouth. A medieval Ethiopian Coptic Church prayer book shows Mary "sprinkling a maiden's eyes with the milk of healing and mercy in a treatment for blindness," no doubt based on breastmilk's ability to cure conjunctivitis.

In many instances, milk is used as a metaphor for purity. "I fashioned their members, and my own breasts I prepared for them, that they might drink my holy milk and live by it," says Christ (Odes of Solomon, 8:14, from early Christian Apocrypha).

In Hebrew scriptures, where the Almighty, or El Shaddai, derives from the word *shad*, meaning "breast," there are also abundant references to milk as a metaphor for goodness and plenty. "In that day the mountain will drip with new wine, and the hills will flow with milk; all the ravines of Judah will run with water" (Joel 3:18).

The confluence of nature's abundance and human milk is echoed in Frida Kahlo's twentieth-century painting *Love Embrace of the Universe*. Here she creates a pantheistic image of Mother Earth, who also has Buddhist and Hindu associations through her posture and four arms. Her left breast drips milk as she holds a "child," Frida Kahlo, who is in turn holding her husband, Diego Rivera, in her arms. It is a powerful melding of diverse pagan and spiritual traditions.

This blurring of boundaries, between cultures, between mother and child, between nature and spirit, and body and emotion, is also touched on in Lilith's fantasy, which follows. Here she shows how friendship and love are also mingled.

Breasts connected the male and female, the physical and spiritual, and the human and divine worlds of Christianity.

—Claire Phillips-Thoryn, "The Sacred Breast"

I had a fantasy once about breastfeeding a friend of mine who was very sad.

It started with his letter. His name is Detritus—not his real name, but appropriate. I have known him since I was nineteen and I lived with my boyfriend in a flat in Bilbao. We were a bunch of young artists with bleak futures. Quite depressing, all of us.

Detritus tried to seduce me, unsuccessfully, every time we were alone. He was and still is very handsome, pale with dark hair and black eyes that have a very special way of looking at my mouth.

But I was not attracted to him. I had a boyfriend at the time, and I am loyal to my boyfriends.

Then he married an American woman he met in New York, and moved with her to Hartford, Connecticut, just about a year before I came here. And since then we have seen each other at only a very few special occasions. But we write each other often.

Many years ago, when he was perhaps only eighteen, Detritus had a vasectomy. His hate for life is so profound that he doesn't understand how people can still be bringing more people into this world. So when I had my baby, I thought Detritus might never write me again. Of course I was wrong, because I soon got a letter from him. He is a very good friend of mine, after all.

He congratulated me, observing the whole protocol about wishing me health and beauty and all that. And then he told me that he was going through a crisis. He had broken up with a girl he loved (he divorced his American wife a while ago), and was not painting anymore, nor writing, and the only thing he could think of that would make him feel better was a sip from my alive milky breasts.

Since then I have this image haunting me. Detritus is crying and I am pulling up my shirt and offering my breast to calm his sadness. It extends into other images that I have seen, or perhaps dreamed, before. I imagine Caravaggio's painting of a father in jail being breastfed by his daughter. But it is not quite that. I don't know how we got to this point, or how the scene may end, or develop. It is a silent snapshot.

The image I see is not sexy, it doesn't turn me on. It is transcendental, and full of meanings, like the Great Mother consoling all her suffering Children. Or the Holy Milk that purifies all our hate and desperation. This is not a sexual fantasy. It is to think that one is able to erase the pain of another's breast with one's own. It is all about calming the sadness, and the hunger, and the hate, with the waters of the soul.

God's Gift

‹─∾─›

I learned of the following story, which was later told to me in full by the mother, Shelley Abbott, when visiting the Mothers' Milk Bank at Austin, Texas. Based at the Children's Hospital of Austin, it is one of only six currently functioning in the United States.

The then program director of the Austin milk bank, Jeanne Mitchell, showed me around the premises, explaining how the milk was donated, pasteurized, and stored in freezers, then administered to sick babies in the hospital. Using testing and storing procedures similar to those of blood and tissue banking, the bank also has a strict screening protocol, which ensures that only healthy mothers with a good milk supply can donate. The milk bank's definition of donor mothers is "healthy women who are currently breastfeeding and have surplus milk." Their preference is for mothers of very young babies, partly because women's milk at this time is at its most nutritious and will be tailored to the needs of premature and very young infants, and partly because it is easier to build up a mother's supply in the first few months after giving birth.

While most of the babies receiving milk from the bank are in the hospital due to illness or prematurity, some are in need simply because their mothers can't produce enough milk, and their babies can't tolerate formula, or because the mothers are unwell. It is also given to adult patients with immunodeficiency diseases. There is a small processing charge of $2.50 per ounce, which covers less than the actual cost of pasteurization, testing, and storage. Patients in financial straits are not required to pay.

Informal "kitchen table" milk banks sprang up in hospitals throughout the twentieth century as wet-nursing became less popular. But most of these were closed down, at first gradually, due to lack of hospital demand for human milk in the 1950s, and then swiftly in the 1980s for fear of passing on HIV-AIDS, and hepatitis C. Milk banks in many European countries continued to operate, and Denmark is considered a leader in the field, with its sophisticated screening and documentation processes.

There are no milk banks currently operating in Australia, although breastfeeding rates overall are among the highest in the industrialized world. In addition to the lack of facilities to store surplus milk in women's hospitals, I was told of incidents in maternity wards in Sydney and Melbourne where small amounts of milk stored by mothers in the hospital fridge were thrown away. Whether this was through ignorance, ill will, or lack of space, no one can say.

According to Alison Sparkes in her article "Spare a Drop?" the first English milk bank was established in 1939 at Queen Charlotte's Hospital, London. When quads were born at Saint Neot's in Cambridgeshire in 1935, a matron at

Queen Charlotte's organized for milk to be collected and flown to the babies. Her scheme was successful, so a milk bank was formally established four years later. Today there are thirteen milk banks operating in the United Kingdom.

In America, the first milk bank opened in 1910 at the Boston Floating Hospital. Historian Jan Golden notes that by 1929 there were milk banks in at least twenty American cities. She observes that from around this time until the 1950s, breastmilk became a commodity "that women sold to earn a living. During the 1920s they earned an average of $25 to $100 a month for their milk." Golden argues that as milk banking became less popular, and formula feeding more socially acceptable, milk was no longer paid for, and instead donated by middle-class mothers for free. As late as 1961, the *Boston Globe* could announce: "Mostly College Grads Selling Mother's Milk." And "By the 1980s," writes Golden, "milk banks depended entirely on volunteer donors." This meant that the donated breastmilk was seen less as a commodity and more as a sacred substance given from the heart. Golden shows how this played itself out, in the following anecdote:

> The transformed meaning of breast milk was illustrated in a 1982 newspaper account of the meeting between Lacie Lynette Smith of Oklahoma and the women whose milk kept her alive. Born with a rare allergic condition, Lacie could ingest nothing but breast milk. Her mother, unable to feed her because she took medication, drained "every milk bank we could find." On the verge of running out of milk, she contacted the milk bank of Worcester, Massachu-

setts—one of 30 milk banks then operating in the United States, and one which boasted 275 active donors. The Worcester institution sent Lacie the milk she needed, and at the age of 19 months, Lacie went to New England to meet her benefactresses. One hundred twenty women gathered at the airport to await her arrival. A reporter asked one donor about her thoughts. "I prayed for this baby," she replied, "I just can't wait to meet her." Envisioning the airport tableau, with the assembly of milk donors surrounding the infant protagonist and her mother, we see a commodity transformed into a sacred substance.

Sacred maybe, but breastmilk is also seen as a rich field for scientific research. The many components of breastmilk have still not been fully quantified, and their potential for treatment of both infants and adults is still largely unexplored. One of the more colorful scientific projects is being conducted by Julie Mennella, a biopsychologist at the Monell Chemical Senses Center in Philadelphia. Mennella is working on the effect of mothers' diets on the flavor of breastmilk, and speaks in vintner's terms about the "carrot note" in the milk of mothers who drink carrot juice, and how their babies go on to prefer their Cheerios in carrot juice.

Although feeding sick babies is their primary concern, the large quantity of breastmilk processed at milk banks makes them perfect locations for these kinds of studies. One discovery being investigated around the time of my visit to the Austin milk bank—the increase in protein levels in pooled donor milk—suggests there might be unforeseen benefits to pooling milk from different donors—or, if protein levels need limiting, in maintaining a separation between different donors' milk.

When I spoke with the women at Austin in December 2000, they were excited to tell me about a device called a Milkoscan, which could analyze and quantify the nutrients in any given batch of breastmilk—if not its flavor. Developed originally for the dairy industry, it is an expensive piece of equipment, worth $60,000 to $80,000. But the Austin women were hoping to raise funds to buy a Milkoscan, since it provides reassurance to doctors who are trained in prescribing precisely measured amounts of medication. Although it is widely understood that breastmilk is often crucial in the treatment of sick and premature babies, and that the use of formula with such babies can increase their risk of serious illness by up to ten times, many doctors would be reassured by the knowledge of just how much of each useful property is contained in the breastmilk their tiny patients are receiving. As Dr. George Sharpe, neonatologist at the Children's Hospital of Austin, put it, "Human breast milk is really as important to these babies as antibiotics are."

In the following story, neither breastmilk nor antibiotics could save Shelley Abbott's baby. Nevertheless, the grieving mother was hopeful of saving others by donating her milk to the Mothers' Milk Bank at Austin.

The connection between grieving and breastfeeding goes back to paintings of the *Mater Dolorosa,* or Grieving Madonna, and no doubt predates these images by many centuries. In one of the questionnaires I received, this image was given a contemporary makeover by a woman who had suffered three miscarriages and uterine cancer and had been told she would "be lucky to have any children at all." She wrote about the closeness and joy of breastfeeding the child she was ultimately blessed with, but wrote, "I also grieved in that time, but in a pleasurable, opening up kind of way. I grieved for the babies that had died, for my own body's illness, and the lessons that cancer had taught me, and for the potential future babies that I didn't think I would ever have. I seemed to spend hours feeding, smiling, crying, and enjoying. It was a sensual meltdown."

In response to my questionnaire the writer Anna Maria Delosso recalled a scene concerning her own mother, in which grief and reassurance similarly came together. "My memories of my mother's breasts involve great blue-veined and creamy breasts being milked by her, by hand, into the bath after miscarrying a child. A time of great sorrow for her, but my child's view of it, at around four or five years old, was as of an outpouring—there was something very reassuring about the milk that would not be needed pouring into the bath, unable to be stopped by drugs or doctors."

Another woman recalled how her mother had a breast removed due to cancer at the age of fifty. As she lay on the operating table in great distress, she consoled herself with memories of feeding each of her children on that breast and focussing on the goodness it provided. Yet another woman emailed to say how she'd nursed her mother, who was ill with breast cancer, and how this had bonded them more closely than before, as the daughter tended her mother's diseased, weeping breasts.

The subject of grief and breasts is yet to be much explored, even though eyes for nipples, and tears for milk, have so often stood in for one another in art and literature, encapsulated in the idea of "expression." There is also a physiological link between the two, as the dip in estrogen causing the postpartum "third-day blues" is a change that allows the milk to come in. As one lactation consultant told me, "I encourage my patients to welcome the change in mood, because when the tears flow, so does the milk."

Note

The Mothers' Milk Bank at Austin is a nonprofit organization supported by grants, donations, and volunteer workers. If you are interested in donating milk, money, or time to the milk bank, information can be found at their website: www. mmbaustin.org.

Other milk banks in the United States are located in Denver, Colorado; San Jose, California; Newark, Delaware; and Raleigh, North Carolina. The Denver milk bank has a special supply of breastmilk for lactose-intolerant babies. There are also milk banks in Canada and Mexico. Further information can be found at the Human Milk Banking Association of North America's website: www.hmbana.org, or by calling (303) 869–1888.

For information on milk banking in the UK, call the United Kingdom Association for Milk Banking at 0208 383 355.

As honey dips from the honeycomb of bees, And milk flows from the woman who loves her children, So also is my hope upon Thee, O my God.

—Odes of Solomon, 40:1, from the Apocrypha

My husband and I have a daughter, Erica Lynn, who was born in 1996, and on June 6, 2000, we had another daughter. We named her Lauren Elizabeth.

She was born with an enclosed hernia on her hip, which really wasn't any immediate threat, but her doctors knew right away she would need surgery. That afternoon we went to Indianapolis, and she had surgery for her hernia that night. While she was being operated on, they also found that her appendix had ruptured about a week prior to her birth. But she was not ill from that; she never had an infection; she was never sick.

We were at Riley Children's Hospital in Indianapolis for five days, and Lauren recovered quickly. She was a beautiful baby. But on November 1, just a few days before she would have been five months old, she became ill. She had a fever of 103 degrees, but we didn't think it was anything severe. That's a pretty good fever, but nothing life-threatening. She was ill on and off all evening. She threw up once, and didn't want to nurse, so we just thought she had the stomach flu. I had called the doctor and asked what to do, what I had to watch for. They weren't all that concerned, and neither was I.

During the night her fever subsided, but by the morning she had a fever again. I called the doctor at 7:00 A.M., and they told me to bring her in first thing, so I took her in before nine, and in that short amount of time—between seven and nine o'clock—she became seriously ill.

She had started breaking out with what I thought was a rash, around her mouth, in the fifteen minutes I was in the waiting room. It was blood vessels breaking in her face. When I took her to the doctor's office and we stepped into the examining room, he said, "Let's go to the emergency room now."

The emergency room at the hospital was virtually across the road from the doctor's office, but within half an hour of being in the emergency room, Lauren's condition had become a life-threatening one. Lauren was diagnosed with bacterial meningitis. She lived for just twenty-four hours after being admitted to the hospital.

They told me that it was streptococcal meningitis, which is the same bacteria that causes strep throat. It's everywhere, there are just different strains of it. It's the leading cause of ear infections. She could have picked it up in the grocery store. It could have been something that might have been on me, from being in somebody else's house, with their children. It could have been anything. She basically just breathed at the wrong time, as one nurse explained to us.

Even before they knew what type of meningitis it was, they were treating her for the worst type. And they suspect, because she didn't respond to the medication, that there might have been something wrong with her immune system.

I questioned this. She was three days shy of being five months old when she died, and she'd never had even a sniffle. They said it could be because I was nursing, and the child's immune system doesn't usually kick in until four and a half to five months. So if the baby happens to get sick right then, it could be like they have no immune system.

We'll never know that for sure, but it was what they suspected. The first time she got sick was just too much.

There's a new vaccine available for meningitis now, but Lauren kind of slipped through the cracks with that. She was born in June, and the vaccine, called Prevnar, became available here in the United States in July or August. It wasn't being given routinely because it was still going through approval and I don't think it was government funded. After Lauren died, many parents in our town were in a panic. It seems everyone was rushing their child to the doctor's office to get the shot, which was being offered for free. Lauren became the "poster child" for meningitis in our area. But whether the shot would have helped her or not if she had a poor immune system, we'll never know.

Lauren became sick on Wednesday night, and died on Friday at noon. I had continued pumping breastmilk all the while she was sick. She wasn't interested in nursing, and I was becoming uncomfortable, so I would go ahead and pump. In the twenty-four hours she was in hospital, I was pumping and trying to store some of the milk. Even though we knew she was gravely ill at that time, a little voice inside of me was saying, "Go ahead and pump. You need to pump." And I guess at the time I thought, "Well, God's telling me I need to pump because she's going to get better." And so I continued.

The first couple of days after she died were a complete and utter shock. My body quit making so much milk, and I wasn't eating much or sleeping well at night. But I was still producing some milk, so I was having to pump at least a couple of times a day. And every time I'd pump, and go to pour that milk down the drain, it just killed me. It was so sad for me because I'd been doing this and storing the milk for so long. I'd done the same for Lauren's older sister, Erica, as I'd worked full-time after she was born and continued breastfeeding. It was so much part of my routine to pump, put the milk into containers, freeze it, and label it. I called it my "liquid gold." Whenever I'd pour it down the sink, I would start crying. And I thought, I can't do this.

I think it was almost a week after she died, and I'd been pumping a small amount, just enough to prevent engorgement, and I thought my milk supply had probably gone way, way down. I asked my doctor about a drug that could dry me up so I could stop pumping because it was so emotionally painful.

Two days after Lauren's funeral, I was in the shower and felt my milk letdown; and it was then that I remembered about the milk bank. I'd read about milk banking when I was looking on the La Leche League's website a few weeks earlier. I'd been looking for advice because my milk supply had been lower than usual, and I contacted a league member. She told me that the birth control pill I was on was the wrong one, so I went off it. Soon after I stopped taking the pill, my milk supply increased.

When I was looking at the La Leche League site there was a link to the Human Milk Banking Association's website, so I looked it up. I'd gone there looking for information about storing milk because I had quite a lot of it. When I saw the pictures of how they store the milk, I was intrigued.

And so it came back to me, there in the shower. I thought, "I fed my baby, why not feed somebody else's?" I knew that the milk bank needed milk for premature infants and for research, and I just thought about it for a day or two, wondering whether to donate my milk and to keep pumping.

There were a couple of things motivating me. I really thought that it was a neat thing I could do. The milk I had for Lauren was a gift from God. I wouldn't have had that gift without her, and this was something I could do to continue her memory. I couldn't stand the thought of pouring all her milk down the drain. So I called the Austin milk bank, which was the one I'd noticed as being listed on the website, and told them about my situation. They told me they needed milk and were more than helpful to get me set up. They were glad to take my donation.

To me, my milk was a part of Lauren that, I guess selfishly, I felt I could keep. It was a part of her I didn't have to give up yet. I loved nursing. I loved the feeling of the letdown, the tingling warmth, the relaxation. I loved giving milk. When Lauren died, I wasn't anywhere near ready to wean her. Being able to continue, with a sense of real purpose, was crucial to helping me heal and overcome my grief.

Once I made the decision that I was going to pump, and that I was going to donate my milk, it was like something clicked. I was emotionally changed. When I knew that I wasn't making milk for my baby anymore, but that I was making milk for other babies, it gave me a kind of hope, something positive to look at, I guess. I knew that I was giving a gift, so I didn't feel so sad, or distraught, as I knew my milk was going to somebody.

It had been difficult to pump right after Lauren died. I would pump as little as I could, as infrequently as I could, just for relief when I became too full. I was basically trying to dry myself up. But once I made the decision to donate, I began pumping every hour or hour and a half, so that over a period of a week or two my supply increased again. It took about a month to get back to what I had before, which was between eight and twelve ounces a day. I'd usually pump about two ounces off, then a couple of hours later I'd pump another two ounces off, and gather it up through the day. I didn't think it was a lot, but the milk bank told me it was wonderful.

After having both my children, I had continued working and breastfeeding, so I was used to pumping. I'm a speech pathologist, and can set my own schedule, as I'm self-employed. So I could feed my baby, then go to an appointment or two, and be back in a couple of hours to nurse again. My mother looked after both my children after we moved back to our hometown. Sometimes she would have to feed the baby a bottle of expressed milk before I'd get back, so I'd just pump instead. It had worked out well when I was consulting full-time, because they had a refrigerator, and I had a private office. So I did a lot of pumping.

As the children became older, it was harder for my schedule, and often we would be out of synch, so I'd do a lot of pumping throughout the week. I'd pull off to the side of the road and pump. I used a nonelectric hand pump so I could pump anywhere. I was pumping in my van, in other people's houses, and everywhere else. When I came home from work, the first thing I'd do was pump, just wherever I was. I'd be preparing a meal with one hand and pumping with the other, returning phone calls, putting clothes away, or whatever I needed to do. It was part of my routine. I basically walked around with the breast pump attached to me!

At one stage I wasn't having much luck with the breast pump, and

I started hand expressing. I had better luck with that, and became quite efficient at hand expression. I had tried it before and didn't have a whole lot of luck with it. But for some reason, maybe because I had nipples of steel, it worked. By then I'd been pumping my breasts for five months; they could have been pinched with pliers and I don't think I would have noticed.

It gave me something to talk about, the fact that I was still pumping after my baby was gone. It helped me to be able to talk about Lauren. People were very curious about what I was doing. Some people thought it was odd enough that I was nursing and pumping, even when Lauren was still alive. I've talked to a lot of women who've nursed and a lot of women who've had trouble pumping or don't want to mess with it.

Storing the milk was something I was used to as well. At first I used plastic bags that are specially made for storing breastmilk. Then the milk bank sent me four-ounce plastic bottles that are sealed and sterilized. When you open them you break the seal and you know it's a clean bottle. That's what I stored most of the milk in. I'd label the bottle with an identification number, the date it was stored, and how many ounces were in the bottle. Then I'd store them in the freezer until it looked like I could fill a carton, which was about fifty or sixty of the four-ounce bottles. About once a month, I sent a carton. I was sending it from Indiana to Texas, which is quite a distance. I would wrap each bottle individually in newspaper, so it was insulated; then I'd put it in the box with five frozen ice packs, in layers around the milk. I'd usually stuff it as full as I could with milk, and then stuff newspaper around that, then tape the box shut. It was sent at the milk bank's expense—they paid for the boxes and milk bottles and shipping.

I felt glad that my milk was going to sick babies who really needed breastmilk and might not do well on formula. But at one point I almost gave it to a baby in our area. My mother knew a woman who was adopting a baby, and told her what I was doing with the milk bank. The woman asked my mother about getting breastmilk from the milk bank for her baby. She was curious about how much it would cost, and whether she could even get milk from them. It's very expensive. If there's a medical need, some insurance companies will cover it—it's $3 an ounce, like liquid gold literally! But I let the woman know that if she was interested in breastmilk, I would donate mine for her baby.

I can't say what her reasons were for not wanting to use my milk. Probably a multitude of things. But I was concerned, too, about possible liability. If for some reason the baby got sick, I didn't want to be held responsible. There wasn't any way that the illness Lauren had could be transmitted through my milk to another baby, but my only thought was, What if the baby gets sick, and then the only thing we'll be able to think about is, well, my baby died. . . . Will they think it's because of my milk? Would they try to sue me? All these things went through my head. I was still willing to donate my milk to this healthy little boy. But she decided to go with formula instead, which I can understand.

I continued donating to the milk bank for the next five months. Then on April 1, 2001, I learned that I was pregnant. I didn't know whether I should continue to pump or not, because of my nutritional needs. But my husband, Rick, and I just felt that in my baby's best interest, and mine as well, I should stop. The milk bank supported my decision.

Even if I hadn't become pregnant, I probably wouldn't have gone on for much longer. My husband was very supportive. He would never have suggested that I stop. He said, "You do that for as long as you need to." He knew it was part of my healing process, but I'm sure at times he became aggravated.

It was getting a bit aggravating for me sometimes too. If I wanted to keep my supply up, I needed to pump four times a day during the day, for about fifteen minutes at a time. And sometimes it wasn't really convenient for me to stop and pump right then! I'd be out shopping, and I would need to pump, so I'd have to interrupt whatever I was doing. I think Rick was beginning to feel that it was a bit inconvenient too.

I was elated at the fact that I was pregnant, but I felt sad when I packaged up the last carton of milk for Texas. I realized it was another stage in letting go of Lauren, of saying good-bye.

I got a call one day from a woman who had lost her baby and was donating milk. We were connected through the milk bank. It turned out that her situation was a little different than mine. Her baby was about the same age as Lauren when he died, but he never got to drink any of her milk because he had a stomach disorder and couldn't keep food down. He was on an intravenous solution. But she had pumped for four months and had stored all her milk, hoping that one day he would get better. After her baby died, she donated all her stored-up milk, in one lump sum. She didn't continue to pump after that, and I can respect that. I wouldn't condemn anyone for not doing what I did. What I did was right for me. It was a very personal decision.

I don't know of anyone else who has done what I've done. I'd love to speak to women who are considering doing this. Because I know it really helped me, to know I was helping someone else.

You know, if there's a mother who called the milk bank just days after her child died and was contemplating doing this and wanted to talk to somebody, I'd like them to say, "Well, you can talk to this person. She's been in your shoes."

Postscript

After Lauren died, Shelley and Rick Abbott set up a foundation in their daughter's name, asking people to donate money to a memorial fund. The money will go to support milk banking, and to raise awareness about meningitis and the vaccine. They are also hoping to set up a scholarship for pediatric nurses. If anyone would like to donate money, please send a check or money order to:

Lauren E. Abbott Memorial Fund
C/o The Northern Indiana Community Foundation
PO Box 807
Rochester, IN 46975

Cost per Liter

If you could buy breastmilk by the liter from the corner store, how much would it cost?

$2.65.

No idea!

$10.

I imagine buying breastmilk would be like buying wine.
     You'd need a testing panel to rate it and price it accord-
     ingly, because each batch is so different and individual.

$20. A steal.

Thousands.

Less than it is worth.

A fortune!

$3.

I think human breastmilk should cost about $10,000 a liter
     given the tortuous way it is expressed.

$50 at least. But wait. If it were going to a baby, it would be
     cheaper than whatever formula costs, to encourage a
     mother to buy it instead.

Priceless.

Relatively inexpensive, even though it's worth its weight in
     gold, because the health department would sponsor it.

$100.

It should cost at least triple what formula costs, but because
     of the Western world's squeamishness about breast-
     milk, it would be the cheapest option, and the poor

women providing it would be the poorest of the poor, selling some part of themselves in order to give their children an education.

$24.95.

$1,000.

$200.

Free. Like love.

I imagine it would be regulated like cows' milk to be the same price as infant formula.

$15.

Breastmilk should never be sold.

One million dollars.

More than a good bottle of wine, say $40. It would be presented in tall, slim, elegant bottles and would be served at room temperature in crystal liqueur glasses.

$4.

Breastmilk is for babies.

$5.

It should cost even less than cows' milk considering how many women are breastfeeding at any given time.

$8.

Four million dollars.

Answer

According to the economist Julie Smith, breastmilk is worth approximately $50 a liter. Based on 1992 Australian figures, Smith estimates that Australian women produced 33 million kilograms, worth $2.2 billion to the economy, which is about 0.5 percent of the GDP. Since 1993 Norway has included human milk output in its annual reports on national food production. It is the only country to do so.

Pressure

T o adopt the dictum that "Breast Is Best" is not always a simple, blouse-unbuttoning process. And within breastfeeding advocacy circles it can sometimes be too easy to dismiss as ignorant or misinformed the large population of mothers who choose not to breastfeed. While this might in some cases be true, it is important to understand the multitude of pressures—practical, physical, and psychological—that might also be influencing these women.

As one respondent to the questionnaire noted, "The pressure on women is profound. I did not like feeding, and comments indicating disapproval were commonplace. Including one from a man who, not unkindly, said, 'You're obviously just not a natural mother!' Nothing could be further from the truth, as I took to motherhood like a duck to water. (Not to mention the fact that I produced plenty of milk and fed my children easily!) The comment angered me—but my anger dissipated somewhat when some months later his wife had a baby and whispered in my ear that she too disliked breastfeeding! . . . We are not given the 'rules' about breastfeeding, but when we break them we are most certainly reprimanded!"

In her book *At the Breast: Ideologies of Breastfeeding and Motherhood in the Contemporary United States,* Linda Blum painstakingly untangles the many conflicting meanings that breastfeeding holds for women of different classes and races in America. She suggests that for African-Americans, for example, breastfeeding has strong negative associations with slavery, since white landowners frequently handed over their offspring to be wet-nursed by black slaves. These women were forced to breastfeed the slave owner's children, often at the expense of their own. In Australia, for different reasons, urban Aboriginal women rarely breastfeed, and those who do only continue for a month or two. As Dana Raphael and Flora Davis wrote in their 1985 study, *Only Mothers Know,* "The poorer the family, the more limited the feeding choices available to her."

For many people, black and white, breastfeeding also continues to be stymied by an image problem. Advocates are seen as overzealous and antisex, as if the cultural infection that blights feminist organizations has spread to those that also promote the traditional practice of motherhood. Although a woman might seek advice over the telephone from a breastfeeding association or La Leche League counselor, many balk at identifying with what they see as these groups' fanatical members.

A UK survey on the media's approach to breastfeeding was reported to *The British Medical Journal* in November 2000. Writing up the results in the *London Times,* Thomas Stuttaford concluded that "breastfeeding gets little positive media coverage" and "is portrayed as a cranky, middle-class habit." He writes, "The researchers suggest that the media by its coverage encourages the belief that 'ordinary families' no longer breastfeed for any length of time, and that breastfeeding is associated with middle-class or celebrity status."

At the same time, the growth of the lactation consultants' profession has created concern among some women that there has been an overmedicalization of breastfeeding, which not only pathologizes the subject, but risks leading to the perception of there being a right and a wrong way to nurse. As Blum also notes, among white professional mothers who return to work as soon as possible after giving birth, breastfeeding has attained an iconic role, proof of a woman's status as a good mother. This is reinforced by images used in advertising for workplace breast pumps, and harks back to the old bogie of the "Supermom," sailing through her day without a wrinkle in her blouse or smudge of her eyeliner. Such developments can lead to the creation of unforeseen and oppressive orthodoxies, which can further put women off breastfeeding.

In her book *The Mask of Motherhood: How Mothering Changes Everything and Why We Pretend It Doesn't*, Susan Maushart records the reasons of women who, even though comfortably middle-class, have chosen not to breastfeed. These range from pain, tiredness, and feelings of incompetence to a reluctance to feed in public, a need for physical autonomy from the baby, a feeling of being "overwhelmed" by the baby's needs, resistance by the baby to the breast, and the mother's wish to share more of the feeding with the child's father. Writes Maushart, "The reality of the breastfeeding experience is that it is as diverse as any other human relationship. . . . There is no doubt that, for many women, breastfeeding does feel natural and joyous and 'empowering.' Yet for at least an equal number, breastfeeding feels more like hard work for which there is little apparent reward."

In this story, a first-time mother reveals what is going through her own mind as she grapples with her fears and struggles to decide what to do.

All things being equal, breast milk is best for babies. Yet all things are not equal, not by a long shot.

—Susan Maushart, *The Mask of Motherhood*

I enjoyed my stay in the hospital, I must say. I was in for seven days because I had a cesarean. I was forty weeks, and I just went to the hospital for my normal visit, with my husband, and my doctor said, "If you want, you can go another week; otherwise I can do it today." He said, "You go and have a chat about it, and don't eat anything." So Mark and I had a chat, and I rang up my mom, and she said, "Yeah, I think you should." I was really scared, but everything was lovely, and the nurses were wonderful. I didn't want to leave in the end. I didn't want to go home!

I think I always had at the back of my mind that I wanted to bottle-feed. I'd seen other women breastfeeding, and it never really turned me on, so to speak. I never thought, Wow, I'm going to do that when I have a baby. I just thought, I'll do the bottle-feeding. And when I went into the hospital, I was more worried about what was going to happen, about the procedure, and the surgery. When they were prepping me for the ordeal, one of the nursing sisters said, "Are you going to breastfeed or bottle-feed?" I looked at Mark and I said, "I've really got no idea. I don't know." And she said, "All right, you think about it, and you decide."

After the ordeal, she was back in the room, and I had to make up my mind. I said, "I'll give it a go and see how I go with it." So that night, I didn't sleep at all, it was awful. They brought Emily in at about three o'clock, and I was in a lot of pain, and I didn't really register what I was doing. They helped me, because I had all the tubes in me. Then in the morning they brought Emily in again, and the thing I panicked about the most was when they left me. They said, "Just yell out if you need any help, and we'll come back," because they had to go and see other people.

They stayed to help the first night, because I didn't know what to do, but the second night, I started to worry. I did try breastfeeding once when the nurse was out of the room. Emily had come off, and then she got back on, and I thought, Maybe I *can* do this. But no, she came off again and she cried, and I started to get stressed. I was thinking, I don't like this, I don't like it. This is going to be too hard for me.

The way the midwives were handling Emily was a little bit on the rough side, too. They weren't doing it intentionally, they were just showing me what to do, and her poor little eyes were just bulging. I felt quite sad, because she was getting shoved on, almost roughly. That was after three days, and I started to crack up under the pressure.

We just both weren't getting the hang of it. We both weren't.

The lady in the room opposite persisted the whole time, and I'd hear her baby screaming, and I'd see her struggling sometimes. I'd pass her in the ward and she looked so tired. She came over to my room and had a little chat, and told me she was really worn out. Emily was the best baby in the hospital. I'd pick her up from the nursery each morning, and they'd say, "She gets a star, she has been so good all night." I saw what some of the women went through, and I'd just think, It's got to be easier to bottle-feed.

I didn't like the feel of it either. It was more of a bitey feeling, like getting nibbled at. When it was happening, I'd be looking at her and she'd be looking at me, and I just felt uncomfortable. I didn't feel relaxed at all.

But my main concern in the hospital was the fear that I might get stuck once I got home. I just thought, What if I got into trouble, if she couldn't latch on, she'd be screaming her head off, and I'd be crying. I'd picture all this, and think, No way, I'm not going through that.

I'm the type of person who needs to know everything and get everything organized beforehand. I always think in the future, so come the third night I was really worried what people would think if I decided to bottle-feed. I was really scared what Mom would think. I thought she might say, "You should give it a go." So I rang her up. I was quite upset and she said, "Now what's wrong, tell me." I said, "I don't know what to do, to breastfeed or bottle-feed, and I'm really depressed about it." She said, "Hey, it's up to you, you do what's best for you. You weren't breastfed, and nor were the others. So don't be worried what I'm going to think. You do what's best for yourself." That made me feel heaps better. Then I rang Mark, and he said, "Whatever you decide, I'm with you, I'm there." He's such a fantastic person. Then one of the sisters was coming on duty and she was so nice. I was so upset. She sat on the bed and had a little chat with me. She said when she met me, she had the impression that I had it in the back of my mind that I wanted to bottle-feed. And she said, "If that's what makes you feel more comfortable, that's what you should do." I felt much better after that, and that's when I started giving Emily the bottle.

But I thought as long as she got the colostrum before I stopped, that would be good, because the colostrum is very good for little ones. So she got the colostrum and that made me feel better. And the nurses were great. A lot of hospitals say, "You'd better breastfeed." I've heard a lot of cases where women are pressured to breastfeed; they don't like the bottles at all.

The last night I was in the hospital, Mark and I went out to dinner. The nurses mind the baby and give you a night out. When we came back, and Mark had gone, I was just getting into my jammies, and my breasts were like cement, with lumps in them. They were rock hard, with pains shooting through them. I quickly went to the nurses, and they said, "That's probably happened because your milk is drying up. We'll have to get you some cabbage leaves."

I had to wear them for a good three to four weeks, twenty-four hours a day. When we got home I had to send Mark down the shop to get a cabbage, which we then put in the freezer. My mom had to help me get dressed. I had to wear a bra all the time, and I felt like I'd been in a war, I tell you. My stomach had to be dressed every day and cleaned with an alcohol swab, and then I had to put on the cabbage leaves. Some hospitals give you tablets, apparently, and they used to use injections to dry up milk. But the nurses thought cabbage leaves were best.

Mark would hold them while I put my bra on. Two big leaves on each side. Every morning after I had my shower, I put fresh ones on.

And again at night. When you put the cabbage leaves on, they stay cold, but only for an hour or so. And the next morning they were soggy and I'd have to peel them off. They were gross. But then I'd get nice cold fresh ones.

When Emily first came home, I felt very secure. I'd prop myself up with the pillows, and hold her face, and she'd touch my face, and I just thought, Oooh. I'd look at her hands, and she'd look at me. I was totally transfixed. I thought that was lovely, her staring at me, and I'd be stroking her little hands. I'd have the bottle, and I'd cuddle her afterward, and she'd go to sleep while we were sitting on the lounge. I'd say, "Wave good night to Dad over there." She'd look at him, and lie on my shoulder.

I felt more confident with the bottle. It's something that comes with instructions, so to speak. I like things that have instructions, that are there in front of me, so I know I'm doing the right thing. And I know I'm getting the advantage, so I feel I get a tick for bottle-feeding. The fact is that you have to do it right, with breastfeeding; otherwise they're not going to get anything. I don't want to hassle around. I'd rather for her to have the bottle, and have her milk. And I wanted to go through the whole thing unhelped and unaided. I wanted to be able to do this.

I also thought, What if my milk dried up, what would I do? I just couldn't go through all the drama. What if the baby dehydrated? Say something happened, maybe an accident, and when I got home she couldn't latch on? Or if I had an accident? How do I handle that? And how do I know when she's had enough? Or she might be getting too much. Or become allergic to it. I would not want that happening to me.

I don't have any regrets. Emily's going to grow up the same as if I was breastfeeding. Most of the mothers in my group did breastfeed, and one still does, but it never got me down. I just thought, Bottles are the best thing. Like they'd be saying, "Well, you've got to steril-ize them and heat the milk," but that never bothered me. We had the procedures when we got home, and we got a sterilizer, and I thought, Breastfeeding may be easier, but bottle-feeding is easy too. It doesn't take long to wash bottles.

Mark and I both liked the idea that he could feed too, that this was his bonding time with Emily. He'd come home from work, and that's when he'd give her the bottle. That made me feel happy within myself that he was bonding with his daughter, because I had her dur-ing the day, and he could do it at night. I was glad that other people could do it as well, like my mom and dad. It makes her less clingy, so she'll go to other people. It made me feel a bit freer.

She's fourteen months old now, and she's on cows' milk. She has a bottle in the morning and a bottle at night, and some juice during the day. She loves it. And since she's been born she hasn't shown any allergy signs, even after immunization—nothing.

I've wanted to have a baby for a long, long time. I was never a career person. I've always been maternal, and I always said I'd love to have a baby since I was eighteen. But I'd see women in shopping centers breastfeeding, and I'd think, I couldn't do that. I'd be too embar-rassed. The other day I was at Westfield Shopping Center, and I glanced at a woman who was feeding her baby in the food court. I just thought, Oh, no way, there's a mother's room, she should be there. I know there isn't anything wrong with it, but I think that's something you should do privately with your little one, not out in the open. I think they're a little bit indecent. And the mothers' room at Westfield's is great. It's got a TV in it, and a microwave.

It's just me, I suppose. I wouldn't like people staring when they went past. I saw a lady once in the supermarket walking around breastfeeding. Some shoppers told the manager, and she was asked to leave. She was around the fruit area. I don't see it as a really big deal. I don't think anyone's going to catch anything. But I don't think what she did was right. Not in the middle of a supermarket. I just think people should be in the right place at the right time.

If it was me, and I was breastfeeding a baby and we were shopping, I would just wait till I went home. If I was on a bus, I'd think, I'm only going to be ten or fifteen minutes away from where I'm going, so I'll just wait. Is that terrible?

Even if I had a good body, I wouldn't parade around in next to nothing. I'm a bit reserved. With Mark I'm fine, and I always have been. But when I was little, my sister would say, "What are you shutting the door for?" I'm still like that.

One of my friends has just stopped breastfeeding. I look at her and think, Oh, there's nothing of you. She's so skinny. I'd be saying, enough is enough. Her baby would not eat, and all she wanted was the breast, poor girl! Part of the problem was getting her to drink out of cups. She'd never accept a pacifier either. And her mom kept going, for fifteen months.

I just thought, No way. And I'd look at all the other mothers when they were breastfeeding and think, Oh, I'm glad I'm not doing that.

Hell Ride

P ain is a hot-button issue among breastfeeding women. Some women feel no pain and are affronted by horror stories from well-meaning friends. "It feels like having your nipples sliced off with razor blades" was one gem I was presented with when pregnant with my first child. When I went on to have pain-free breastfeeding, I was bemused that such horror stories were circulating, and wondered if they were part of the formula manufacturers' armory of marketing strategies.

As another woman who also had pain-free breastfeeding wrote in her answer to the questionnaire: "Something that really bothers me about this subject is when I hear or read woman saying that breastfeeding hurts, or at least hurt in the beginning. This can potentially scare off a new mom who might be thinking about breastfeeding. . . . Breastfeeding is delightfully pleasurable and should be so from the beginning!"

The view of lactation consultants is that discomfort at first can be normal but should pass. Any pain is a sign that something is wrong and should be corrected. Yet for women who do experience pain, there don't always seem to be reasons, and there are not nearly enough warnings about what to expect. For these women, the soft-focus advertising for nursing pads and maternity wear must begin to look like a sick joke as they find themselves mopping up blood instead of milk. As one woman with severely cracked nipples wrote, "After a feed, Emilie used to have blood dripping out of her mouth." Another wrote, "Some days, Jonathan took in so much blood with his milk, he did diapers that looked like meconium: black and sticky."

Pus appears too, on occasion. As one woman reported, "When Lucy was about twelve months, I suffered recurrent mastitis in the left breast and ended up in the hospital. I won't go into the details of green pus oozing from my nipple, it was hideous!" But it's not always a disaster. A woman hospitalized for the removal of a breast abscess wrote that this finally helped her to get things right: "The hospital was great, and allowed baby and me to stay in a maternity room so as to get any extra help needed."

Cracked and grazed nipples might seem minor in comparison to mastitis or a breast abscess, but as one woman pointed out, they can in some ways be harder to bear. As one lactation consultant and midwife who'd experienced both wrote: "The pain from cracked or bruised nipples and having to put the baby to the breast is worse than mastitis—probably because it goes on for so long, and it wears you down emotionally."

Even without engorgement, cracked nipples, mastitis, or the fungal infection thrush, all of which are common, many women feel pain from letdown. For some this is a warm and pleasant tingling that passes quickly, but for others it involves stabbing pain, which can be long lasting. Other women experience pain throughout the breastfeeding period, for no apparent reason. And of course, there is nothing quite like being bitten by extra-sharp, newly minted teeth. As a reason to wean, a teething baby ranks high on the list.

Well-meaning professionals glossing over the pain can add to the frustration. As one woman recalls, "The midwife said, 'Breastfeeding shouldn't hurt,' and attempted to show me the basics of good positioning. It didn't help. . . . The next two weeks were a descent into hell. . . . Oh, the grief. Even as I type now, I am crying, three-and-a-half years later."

Several other women noted that the hospital midwives, while helpful, all had different techniques for achieving the perfect latch, adding to the mother's confusion. As one woman, whose summary of difficulty was "pain, pain and more pain," wrote: "Every time I pushed the help button a different midwife would come in with a different technique. I think I was basically in shock that something that seemed so elementary and straightforward could be so difficult."

The psychological effect of pain while breastfeeding can be underestimated, or overshadowed by information about postnatal depression, even though the two can be related. The effect on mental health of a negative breastfeeding experience, where disappointment and a sense of failure are combined with exhaustion and pain, is rarely discussed. Like much else to do with breastfeeding, it is contained within that discreet period of breastfeeding time, and there is little attention paid to it outside mothers' groups. Getting help through initial difficulties can be crucial for the recovery of the mother's self-esteem, and for establishing a loving relationship with her baby. As one woman wrote, "After my bout of mastitis I was in a pit of despair. I thought life couldn't get any worse and I'd made the biggest mistake of my life in becoming a parent. One day as I was feeding, I suddenly realized that there was no pain and looked down to see my son looking at me intensely. I kept looking and he stopped feeding for a moment and gave me the biggest smile. That was the day I finally fell in love with him."

Another respondent pointed out, "I never expected breastfeeding to be so difficult and painful, and unlike giving birth there is no set period of time when the pain will be over. There didn't seem to be any light at the end of the tunnel. Thank goodness, three months into it we seemed to click, and after that it became the natural and beautiful experience I'd always envisioned."

There is also the anguish of what one woman called her "faulty breasts," leading to a difficulty that didn't resolve itself over time. She wrote, "As much as I nursed and pumped (with a new baby who had an excellent suck and latch), the milk I produced was nominal at best. It was terrifying to watch my baby dehydrate and lose weight and to know that the lumps of flesh on my body posing as breasts were really just lumps of flesh and not good for much besides decoration. I worked very hard to achieve a successful breastfeeding relationship with my newborn, and finally—using [a lactation aid]—I was able to breastfeed her to the satisfaction of both of us. But I was still extremely sad about the whole thing. . . . I felt like a fraud in the exercise of life."

In the following story, Annette tells of her grueling time breastfeeding her two sons, where she experienced just about every difficulty in the book. Like others before her, she too encountered contradictory advice, and despaired at the lack of adequate knowledge among many health professionals. And she too hit a wall of pain and fatigue. But with the help of her family, and a resilient sense of humor, she somehow survived the ordeal.

Ordinary . . . women normally discover in the course of things . . . that they have been given a hopelessly sanitized version of the physical travails involved in normal breast-feeding.

—Susan Maushart, *The Mask of Motherhood*

I was looking forward to breastfeeding my second baby because I thought I'd mastered it with Langley, my first child, after quite a long time. I'd been through cracked nipples, and thrush, and figuring out the rhythm, and regulating my supply. I remember breastfeeding in the bedroom, and the milk shooting out across the room. My cousin from London was lying on my bed watching, and the next thing he looked up and the milk hit him on the head. He's gay. And he said, "Oh my God, Nette, that makes me completely sick!" We laughed and laughed.

After all the trials and tribulations of breastfeeding my first baby,

I really felt betrayed, because so much of the advertising I saw about breastfeeding made it look like this natural, easy, painless process. It's as though it was what we were put on earth to do. I remember thinking, This is absolute bullshit. Because for me, after leaving the hospital, it was diabolical.

It was hard for about the first six weeks, which is a difficult time anyway in a woman's life. I'd given up work to have the children, so I had all that emotion of not working and not having the interaction with people I was used to. The social interaction I did have was with people who talked babies and breastfeeding, and I couldn't stand it.

My first big problem with feeding was that I had an overflow of milk. The milk would come out too fast, and Langley would often vomit after I'd fed him. So I went to see lactation consultants, and they'd have me in all these different positions to breastfeed. Lying back with pillows. Rolling on one side. Feeding lying down. I got to the stage where I was leaning way back breastfeeding, trying to stop this fast flow of milk. And then they had me expressing before I breastfed, so I'd get up before each feed and attach myself to the pump, which we called the milking machine.

Then I developed thrush, and a cracked nipple, which was partly caused by my oversupply and the difficulties with attaching properly. So for several weeks it was extremely painful.

My husband, Jeff, became involved, and the whole sexual thing went out the window entirely. Jeff became so interested in breastfeeding—how I was going to do it, and how I was feeling—he would sit up with me every night when I was breastfeeding. It was a big effort on his part, and it was amazingly helpful. He was under a lot of stress at work, but he just made it his project. And if Mom was here, she'd come in and she'd sit with me too.

Mom and Jeff were really probreastfeeding, and everyone I seemed to speak to, at the clinic, at the hospital, anywhere I went, was really a bit pushy for me to keep breastfeeding. I wasn't ready to give up, but there were a couple of times with Langley when I thought, This is unbelievably hard, I think it would be easier on a bottle. But I was committed. I phoned the Breastfeeding Association, and some of their advice wasn't in the reality of living, like some of the positions they suggested to breastfeed and how often I should feed.

Sometimes it was funny, sometimes it was outrageous, but most of the time we agreed that breastfeeding was a pretty hard process.

Finally with Langley it all came together, and I fed him for six months, and then I continued giving him two feeds a day until he was nine months old. The only reason I gave up was that I got an abscessed tooth and started antibiotics, and I didn't want him to be exposed to the drugs. So I got back onto the milking machine, and weaned him. He was basically quite happy to do that, and I was happy, and that's how it ended.

I'd finally mastered breastfeeding and I was really looking forward to the second experience. I felt confident about breastfeeding. I enjoyed it and the convenience. I thought it was a great start to life, with the protection it offered to the baby. I thought I'd keep on doing it.

Well, the second experience was absolutely horrific. It all started in the hospital. Because I was a second-time mom, there was a bit of an attitude coming from the nurses. It was as if they were thinking, Oh, she's a second-time mom. She's done it before, and I don't need to spend as much time with her. But a lot of mothers I've spoken to have found the second time harder.

I'd also had a rare reaction to the anesthetic for my cesarean, and was suffering incredible pain. I have a one-in-a-million nervous system, which means epidurals don't work on me—as they discovered after the delivery. The whole pain relief process was shocking with Langley, I couldn't stand it. So that was my main concern when Brenton was born, that the epidural wouldn't be painful. But it hurt putting it into my back like you wouldn't believe. Then it didn't work properly, so I could feel them putting on the alcohol swab before making the incision, and I could feel them stitching me up again afterward. Over the next few days, all the extra epidural fluid in my back had to be absorbed. The stitches on the incision were also causing problems, and I'd shiver and shake with the pain. Then I had an allergic reaction to the tape they used to attach the epidural, so my back was raw with welts, and for about two weeks afterward I could barely lie down.

Even though I felt confident about breastfeeding, I thought I just needed a refresher course on attaching. So I asked the nurses if they could take a look at how I was doing, if they had time. I did get some help with attachment, but they left me with taking him off. Brenton would drag the nipple as he came off. I changed my position, but despite concentrating on being relaxed so he could latch on correctly, and me thinking, Yeah, I can do this, I'm very relaxed with breastfeeding, and I don't have my shoulders up to my ears, he'd keep slipping off—and I ended up leaving the hospital with a massive cracked nipple.

Just after we came home, Brenton and I came down with the flu. So in the first week we had Brenton in the hospital. Then at five weeks Brenton contracted bronchiolitis and was in intensive care. He also had sleep apnea, so we needed to monitor his breathing. I was expressing through all this, with a severely cracked nipple. I'd be in the hospital, pumping to keep up my supply; and with my shocking flu, and the cracked nipple, I got mastitis.

I also got thrush on my nipples again because of all the pumping I was doing while Brenton was in the hospital. But I thought, No worries, I've mastered thrush on the nipple, I know what to do.

I called the lactation consultants in again for the mastitis, and one of them told me to use a nipple shield. You listen to all this advice and you just do it, so I had the nipple shield on for too long, and the nipple shield was moist, so it made the cracked nipple worse as well as the mastitis. I remember sitting in the armchair in my bedroom, thinking, This is the most agonizing experience I've ever had.

It was so painful to breastfeed that I would get into a complete sweat whenever I knew it was time for Brenton to latch on. The cracked nipple was really severe and became infected, and then I got it in the other nipple, so I had cracks in both nipples. I was so desperate I phoned up every lactation consultant who was on standby in Sydney. I paid $250 to get someone to visit. She looked at my positioning and propped me up with more pillows, and she said, "Keep going, you'll have to do it."

It was just agony. But I was very committed. I could really see the value—probably from my food industry background. I think it's as good a start as a baby can ever get. But I resented the attitude. It's a bit like they were saying to me, "This is what we have nipples for, and this is what we have breasts for, and that's what we're destined to do if we have children." Everyone kept on reinforcing my view that it was the best thing for the baby.

I'd be sitting up in my bedroom, propped up in pillows, and I had Mom and Jeff with me while I'd attach, and even my brother at one stage. It had become a family affair with feeding. Everyone would visit. Everyone who knows me has investigated my nipples, I'm quite convinced about that. And everyone would look at the cracks and say, "Oh my God!" There was pus in the cracks, and even my brother, who's had kids, and my cousin who was out here could not believe the state of my nipples.

As far as anything sexual is concerned, it was absolutely zero. Everyone was offering support. I think it's the second baby thing again. You're not worried if people see your nipples. You don't care. And everyone knew I didn't care.

Another consultant came in and she was mortified. "Oh my God, I can't believe you're still using nipple shields, that's why you've still got the cracks! You have to attach without using the nipple shields, it's the only way you'll get over it. And your positioning is wrong because of the nipple shield."

I took off the nipple shield, and I tell you, I burst into tears then before I started to feed. I was in floods of tears. And then it all reversed. All of a sudden, all these people who had always supported breastfeeding said, "For God's sake, give up!" Mom was saying, "Give up! You shouldn't be in such a state!" My brother would say, "Bloody hell, Nette, this is just ridiculous." So then I had all this pressure to give up. But I thought, I've come this far, I'm not giving up now!

Of course, at the same time, Langley was going through all this second baby stuff. Every time I went to breastfeed he would do something naughty, the standard kind of things that I don't think are covered a lot in the books. Even if I'd been confident with breastfeeding, I had the demands of someone very jealous about the breastfeeding. It was an entirely new situation. So in many ways, it was not as relaxing and as easy as I thought it would be.

Quite apart from the pain and the hassles, the whole thing had become a huge disappointment. I'd gone into this with the preconceived idea that I'd mastered breastfeeding. I wasn't going to have another baby, so I wanted to squeeze every little bit of juice out of this situation. I was really going to enjoy it. And then I didn't, again. It was far worse the second time. The cracked nipples were worse, the mastitis was there, and the thrush wasn't going away.

I saw so many experts—everyone knows my breasts, I'm quite sure about that. My usual doctor at that time went away on a skiing trip, so I went up to the medical center and got some more wrong advice from there. Every doctor and lactation consultant told me it was thrush. So every second moment spare, I was airing my nipples. When I was still in the hospital with Brenton, I'd lie with the curtains closed, airing my breasts. I used hair dryers. Then I got the last lactation consultant back in, for a massive amount of money. I was so desperate.

She gave me a whole list, from another lactation consultant in Melbourne, of all the things I had to do. Bicarbonate of soda washes, changes to my diet. My only saving grace at this stage was my glass of wine in the night, mind you, and even then I was told no, because of the yeast. I wasn't allowed to eat peanuts, watermelon—tomatoes were even on that list. No bread, nothing with yeast in it. And then I get another list about what I should have. And to sun my nipples where possible. So I'd go through everything, follow this list. But I've still got thrush.

My nipples were red raw. The cracks had finally healed, but it didn't matter, because my nipples were so puffed and constantly itchy, it was extremely painful when Brenton latched on. A nurse suggested using gentian violet, which is an old-fashioned remedy for drying out skin. They don't sell gentian violet in Australia anymore, so I had to comb the earth to find someone who still had some in their shed, or medical cupboard. I eventually found some under my mother's house, which was once my grandfather's. We worked out it must have been twenty years old, but we figured that was the only way we'd get any. So I painted my nipples purple.

The thrush was so aggravating, I could not have anything up against my nipples. Itchy! I couldn't stand the rubbing. So the nurse who had suggested the gentian violet said, "You'll have to get some small plastic tea strainers to protect your nipples."

It's quite difficult to get small plastic tea strainers. You can only get large ones. So Jeff scoured all the local shops to find some. He burned off the handles so we were left with just the strainer, and I started going out with tea strainers over my nipples. I'd be in jumpers to hide the lumps, and it would be unbearably hot. And they'd press down, and I'd come home with these great suction rings around my nipples.

Finally I gave up going out and just let people come and visit me, the aggravation was so bad. We're talking eight, nine weeks here, twenty-four hours a day, of extreme tenderness. We went through three or four different thrush treatments, creams and oral treatments. Nothing worked. I finally took Diflucan, at $35 a tablet. They said, "Well, it's the only thing you can do. One or two tablets should do it." I took four, and there was no change.

So I went back to see my regular doctor, who said, "I'm really concerned about this being diagnosed as thrush. I'm going to get some tests done for you." It turns out there was absolutely no yeast on my nipples at all. The sunning, the gentian violet, had completely dried them out. I had dermatitis. It was probably thrush for the first few days, but those first few treatments would have turned it into dermatitis. And with the diet that I was on, and the bicarb, the airing of the nipples, and all the other treatments that I had tried—all of them were making it worse. If you have dermatitis, you don't expose it to sunlight. So my nipples were sunburned. I'd been lying in the sun to dry my nipples out, thinking it was thrush. That was absolutely universal advice. So I would say to myself, "Will I go out for a coffee, or will I sun my nipples?" And I'd sun my nipples instead of going out and having a break!

This was just before the 2000 Olympics, and my doctor said, "Go and see this dermatologist. She's a mom, and she really has a great understanding of these things." I phoned, and they said, "Sorry, she's booked up because all the doctors are away for the Olympics." Here it was September, and they're saying, "You won't get in until November."

In the end, I begged. "I won't last that long, not until after the Olympics. It's just not possible. I will not last that long!"

I think they thought I was going to kill myself. I was still committed to feeding through all this, but there was this desperation in my voice. The doctor was marvelous. She phoned me back and she said, "Look, I'll come in early, just especially." Then she saw my case and she said straight up, "It's dermatitis of the nipple." I was put on cortisone ointment, with Vaseline to protect my nipples between feeds. It took six weeks to clear up.

I'd had it in my mind that I'd continue to breastfeed Brenton for as long as I'd breastfed Langley, but I couldn't take it anymore. The whole second experience was the worst I can ever imagine. I'd only lasted four months!

Around this time my cat Nooska, who had slept with me for ten years and would sit up with me of a night while I breastfed, then sleep under the bassinet, had to be put down. That was the last straw. I cried for weeks after that.

Then I found a baby bird in the park next door, fallen out of its nest. I'm an animal lover and had nursed lots of animals. I used to work at the zoo at one stage. It wasn't a native bird, so the organization that looks after sick wildlife couldn't take it. So I said, "Okay, I'll look after it."

I remember going out to pick up my mother from the airport. I was driving home when Jeff phoned and said, "Nette, I hate to tell you this, but our cat"—our other cat—"has got the baby bird." Honestly, I lost the plot. I nursed that baby bird like it was my own. I nursed it with treatments and antibiotics, and I cried over that bird.

Then I started to weep over anything. If Brenton did something, or Langley was naughty, I'd just cry and cry.

My mother and Jeff got together after one of my big sessions with the bird, and Mom said, "Nette, you've looked after sick animals before, and we've had a lot of animal deaths. I can't believe you've got yourself into this state. It's just not you. I think you're suffering from depression. You have to stop crying." And I just said, "I can't."

I could not stop crying. I had severe postnatal depression and was prescribed Zoloft. I fed Brenton for a few more days, but I didn't want to expose him to the medication. That was the reason why I finally gave up breastfeeding.

I'd hoped to wean Brenton gradually over a few weeks, but one bottle and he wouldn't go back on the breast. So in the end I got the old milking machine out and pumped, even on my very last days of breastfeeding! And I graciously poured that last milk down the sink.

I laugh now. So much for expectations. Nothing went as planned. I'd had enough. If another drop of milk ever came out of my nipple, I think I'd vomit.

It definitely has changed my relationship with Jeff. I don't feel the same way about breasts and intimacy and being touched on the breasts and the nipple. I think it's because I had so much pain. I don't think it's to do with breastfeeding. And Brenton's just turned one, so we're not talking a long way down the track. I'm sure we'll overcome that. It's a hard call, but I really wonder if I'll enjoy having my breasts touched, and being sucked on the nipple. I just don't think it's going to be the same.

It changed my relationship with Dad too, in a good way. My dad hardly ever visits Sydney, and he's a bit of a traditionalist, very different from Mom. They're both broad-minded, but my dad's quieter, doesn't say a lot, and even he was involved with the breastfeeding drama. At one stage my nipples were so sore and cracked, I sat at the table at a family dinner with no top on, with my painted nipples, and I said, "I'm that desperate, Dad, do you mind?" Everyone else had seen me with my nipples, but Dad hadn't. I remember him coming into the dinner and saying, "Well, this is a first." And here I am, forty years old, at the table, with no top on, and with these bright purple nipples. I thought, This is a family dinner we'll never forget. We should have taken photos. Dad, who I never thought would be exposed to that kind of thing, was fantastic, and it changed our relationship.

Speaking from my experience, I'd say there's a lot of preconceived, incorrect, and totally contradictory ideas about breastfeeding. My mother says I had information overload with the first baby. I'm sure that's a common experience, because you're trying so hard to do everything correctly. There's lots of information about how you attach and how you position, but there's not much about the realistic details, the nitty-gritty of breastfeeding. The rhythms and small, intuitive things.

It's teamwork, to be honest. It takes time for things to really work between the baby and you. The strongest team are the baby and mother, and there's no doubt it takes a while to get that team up and running—it's like coaching, really. And then there are other supportive people around that group, who make a second team. My mother used to stand behind me and hold my shoulders down when I was stressed from the pain. All those people who'd come to see me in my bedroom and rearrange my pillows and sit up with me at night, and they'd reposition me, and I'd take a few deep breaths, and they put a stereo in the bedroom, so I could listen to relaxing music—they were all part of the team.

I give advice to people I know and I say, "For godsakes, get some books, read up about it, it's not all it's cracked up to be. It's really a great thing, and I'm really, really for it, but I tell you, when you get to the hospital you're so tired, and so overwhelmed, and so excited, and there are so many emotions anyway, it's really good for you to know a bit more. Then when the baby arrives, you've got visitors, and the staff at the hospitals just don't have the time to help. And try and sit with someone who can breastfeed."

No one told me that. There's no book that says, "Try to pal up, like in a mentoring system, just like you have in business, where you can pal up with someone who knows what they're doing." I think that's one of the best pieces of advice that I could give to anyone. To actually spend time with a mother who's fully in the rhythm of breastfeeding and is willing to share information. I'd be happy to go on a mentoring program. And I'm sure there are lots of women who would do the same. I'm not really suited to mothers' groups. But I wouldn't mind if there was a system where you could pal up with someone who's a bit like you in age or background, who's really in there, past that first twelve weeks, and they can say, "Well, you know, this is what I've found."

You could go and say, "I'll buy you a cup of coffee, I just need a couple of sessions, while you're feeding." No interruptions with kids running around in parks, or whatever, just a really relaxed place. Then maybe see if you can get together for a meeting after your baby arrives. And if you do form a bond, you can ring later if anything goes wrong.

Sometimes at night, I'd be breastfeeding Brenton, and I'd hold his head and think, His head fits in my hand, just there. They were little things, but I'd try and look at something that was good about it. Often I didn't need to make an effort to do that. And he loved it, through all the mastitis, through everything. It's not that every mother is destined to do it. But I do think it's the closest time you'll ever have with your children.

I laugh now. We all laugh about it. There were times, after I'd finished a feed, where we'd all be together, saying, "God, do you believe this?" But even with the cracked nipple, I said, "Oh it's a cracked nipple, I'll get over it."

I remember thinking, This is just going to be a beautiful experience.

Rain

~~~~~~~~~~~

One of the sections of my questionnaire, to both men and women, concerned breastfeeding and sexuality. The majority of respondents said that there was little change to their sexuality, although many women found it harder, especially in the early stages of breastfeeding, to enjoy having their breasts fondled or sucked as part of foreplay. If their nipples weren't feeling tender, they felt their breasts should be reserved for the baby. And many women were simply too tired to be interested in sex.

Others, who breastfed for longer, gradually included their breasts again; and many men reported enjoying the larger size of their partner's lactating breasts. Some women noticed that their orgasms were stronger when their nipples were being stimulated enough for them to produce milk. Others were simply amused to notice, in reverse, that orgasm caused their breasts to fountain.

For men whose partners are not interested in sex after having children, there is some compensation in being allowed to watch breastfeeding. As one father wrote matter-of-factly: "I had no negative feelings when my wife breastfed our

children. I thought it was beautiful and I loved watching. I
still enjoy watching women breastfeed. . . . I even find it sexually stimulating. I never felt excluded while my wife breastfed, even though, with our second child, our sexual
relationship was not as good."

A small number of men and women reported more than a
passing sexual interest in lactating breasts and wrote about
how they incorporated this into their sex lives, to the extent
that some postponed weaning the baby; or considered inducing lactation just for themselves.

Here is one woman's contribution, based on a relationship without children:

> I once had a boyfriend whose sexual fantasy was to be
> breastfed as part of foreplay. This was the hugest
> turn-on for this guy, and if I even so much as men-
> tioned it he would be beyond himself with desire. I
> never found this odd or offensive and used to indulge
> this fantasy mentally for him during sex. I know that
> he has a wonderful mother and they are very close.
> She is a beautiful and nurturing woman, but it never
> occurred to me to ask him if he was ever breastfed. I
> am not someone who believes you must have a nur-
> turing mother hangup to have this fantasy—far from
> it. Breasts are incredibly sexy and therefore breast-
> feeding is also, for some men (and women).
>
> My ex-boyfriend and I shared this fantasy for a few
> years together, and I know he still has this desire
> because we've discussed it recently as a result of your
> questionnaire. I was never turned on by it personally,

but think it is a beautiful and harmless fantasy that a lot of people probably enjoy in their private times but are too scared to share because it's such a taboo topic—a real shame.

In the past few years several websites have been set up especially to create an Internet community for couples who are interested in adult nursing. Two of the more informative ones, the Society for Nursing Couples, and the Community of Adult Nursing, include detailed instructions on how to induce lactation and what to expect from the breastfeeding partnership. They also post stories and photographs from their members. Although there is a strong sexual element in many of these stories, what is striking are the references to the deepening of intimacy and friendship that an adult nursing partnership seems to create. The overall tone of these websites is not unlike that of a politely earnest bird-watching community. Though explicitly detailed, their function is not necessarily sexual arousal.

Three of the male respondents to my questionnaire confessed to a long history of fantasizing about, and practicing, breastfeeding sex. Several other men contacted me by email anonymously while I was researching this book, seeking information about making contact with lactating women.

One man told me how his desire had taken him by surprise, after accidentally tasting breastmilk when he had a one-night stand with a single mother. He wrote, "After she went home, I was sickened. This did not last, however. The disgust evolved into profound desire by the next week." He then "fantasized about it extensively" before he got married and had children. "Although sex was more infrequent it was more exciting with the addition of lactation, and I felt more intimate with my wife than I ever had before."

Another questionnaire respondent was extremely erudite on the subject, having devoted his spare time to collecting examples of adult nursing in literature, film, and art—perhaps in compensation for the difficulty of finding opportunities in real life to nurse from his partners. He spoke of the way in which breastfeeding "intensified the lovemaking" and described in detail his first experience of nursing as an adult: "The first time it was warm, surprisingly sweet, and slightly musky. As you suckle, the milk changes in texture and body, beginning light and thin, then increasing in richness. It is difficult to describe or to be objective about the taste, or to separate it from the act itself, because it is all part of the total, somewhat overwhelming experience. It is a highly intimate and emotional experience, as well as physical. The quantity of milk consumed is probably small, though the sensation is of mouth-filling richness."

The following story was inspired by some of the anonymous emails I received. Please note that it is sexually explicit, so feel free to skip this story if you might be offended! As the respondent, quoted above, thoughtfully pointed out, "Other, more extreme erotic acts are discussed openly, publicized, and even joked about. But rarely this one. I wonder why."

He went on to answer his own question: "I suspect that adult nursing is a hidden desire of many men and women, many more than will admit to it. On the other hand, I doubt that the desire is overwhelmingly common. . . . The subject is rare in conversation, Internet communication, literature, film, art, erotica, or even pornography. If it were common, even if repressed, I suspect there would be more avenues catering to it. After all, every other whim seems to be readily catered for on the Internet. Opportunity is another relevant factor. If someone has a shoe fetish or a predilection for elbows, just as examples, these whims may be indulged almost limitlessly. By contrast, opportunities for adult nursing, even if both parties are willing, are comparatively rare, limited, or short term."

What follows is one of those rare, in this case literary, opportunities.

I can think of nothing more intimate and erotic than suckling the warm, milk-filled breast of a woman I care deeply for.

—Lecheluver, on the Internet

I love women with big breasts so I can suck them. When I close my eyes I can imagine their soft underbelly squashed against my face, and their hard nipples pressing into me.

I don't feel suffocated, because I imagine I am the one having my tits sucked. I am the one who can squirt fountains of milk when another person is lapping at my nipples. I feel the pleasure of my creamy liquid running in rivulets down my belly, of having my areola gently chewed like soft-baked cookies. I can imagine bursting my banks, until all my hard edges turn soft and wet. It would feel like coming, only for hours and hours.

I am still me, with the woman's milk filling my mouth and spilling down my chin. But I am the woman too, with big leaking breasts that soak through my shirt, and sway as I walk, and turn every head my way.

I have a friend called Lara who is lactating, and she comes to my place sometimes. We had a brief sexual affair years ago, but we've stayed close since then. We love being together, talking about anything—problems at work, how our partners or her children are doing, what we've been reading, who we've been lusting after. We like cuddling, and being close, in a way that drifts between friendship and affection, and sex. Sometimes we kiss and I fondle her breasts, or brush the tangles from her long hair. But mostly we just enjoy being cozy. If it's cold, I light a fire in the grate and lay cushions down so that we can lean against each other on the floor, enjoying the warmth of our bodies, and drinking wine, or reading.

Sometimes nothing more happens and we fall asleep, until Lara realizes she'd better go home. But a couple of times it's been different. If she's feeling relaxed enough, and a bit playful, she'll take off her bra, and fondle her nipples while I'm watching. I keep my clothes on, but she likes to pull up my shirt and stroke my chest, and rub her breasts against me.

At first small drops of thin, bluish fluid ooze from the end of her nipples. She lets them dribble onto my lips, and teases me a bit. It always surprises me how much heat radiates from her breasts as she presses them like pocket-warmers against my face, trying to slow down the drips, while staying just out of reach of my tongue. But her milk flows out anyway, warm and vanillary. This is when I can't stay passive, and lick at her nipples, and fondle her breasts. Then she gets bossy, and asks me to start sucking all the milk out of her. She says her breasts are too full, and she instructs me to suck on them as hard as I can, but to be careful not to bite her.

We lie side by side and I move down to concentrate on my task. I use my tongue to pull as much of her areola into my mouth until her nipple reaches my palate. Her warm doughiness fills me until my lips can't open any wider. It's surprisingly hard work to keep the milk flowing at first, and then it spurts against the back of my throat, making me gag. After that I get into her rhythm and swallow as much as I can. The overflow runs across my face and trickles behind my ears. I can feel her other breast resting against my face, and dripping onto my neck. Even my hair is being rained on. I love being soaked in her warm stickiness, and it encourages me to keep going, even when my mouth is aching from the effort.

I try to reach down to rub her crotch, but she wriggles out of reach, and moves my hand away. I content myself by playing with her other breast, hefting its weight and clamping her nipple between two fingers so that her milk stops dripping down my arm. My grip reminds her that she needs to change sides, and she pushes her second breast into my mouth, making me concentrate on swallowing more milk. She gets bossy again, and tells me in her jokey stern voice to make sure I suck every drop out of her, or else.

Then she starts to come, just from me sucking her breasts. She pulls me toward her tightly, and wraps her leg around my hips, drawing me even closer so that she can rub her clitoris against the outline of my hard penis. Then she arches back and the milk shoots out, spraying all over the cushions, and my face.

I love feeling her relax against me, and we lie there peacefully, listening to the fire, and relishing the sticky mess. As we doze off, I can't help thinking that all this milk everywhere should not be wasted.

Breastspeak

If your breasts could speak, what would they say?

God! Look at us!

I wish we were the same size.

Go away. We're busy.

Have cosmetic surgery, immediately.

Suck me! Relieve the engorgement!

Please try trimming your baby's fingernails more often.

Can you stop that child from biting us now? Please?

Lose some weight, you fat cow. We're sick of being an
   F cup.

Give me a break. I'm tired.

I'm getting old.

Piss those rotten bras off, will you?

Leave me in peace!

How could you do this to me?

Stop giving us such a hard time!

Can't you do something to fix this supersensitive right
   nipple?

Feed me!

Sorry we look so sad and droopy.

Don't worry, we know you would have been lost without
   our support over the last two years. And a child's happiness cannot be measured against the aesthetics of perky
   boobs.

Why have I shrunk? Why can't I be like I was?

Stop complaining. We did our best.

What will we do if you don't have another baby?

Give it a rest, sister!

O ye of little faith. See what we can do. You thought we were ugly and shriveled, but behold, we are full and round and firm and beautiful.

Time to look after *yourself*.

You've done well. Now enjoy your sensuality and be proud of us!

Finally, you appreciate us!

Love me! Caress me! Pamper me!

I love you, you are safe.

Thank you for letting me live my purpose—what more could anyone ask for?

Thank you for trusting us and yourself.

We are beautiful, we are sexy, and we have served our role extremely well.

Look after us. We're important.

I am having a break, at last.

Thank you for all that lovely sucking.

I will miss it when it's gone forever.

Love me, and remember my abundance. Revel in the sensations that travel through me still, and don't ever feel ashamed of my slow droop.

Adopting Elizabeth

In Laura Esquivel's novel *Like Water for Chocolate*, the teenage virgin Tita puts her hungry baby nephew to her breast and is amazed to discover that she can feed him. This has often been interpreted as magical realism, yet it's not so implausible as all that. Women can induce lactation without becoming pregnant, though this is not well known.

It is also not well known that a woman can continue lactating beyond menopause. Historians of wet-nursing such as Jan Golden have recorded how some wet nurses continued producing milk into their eighties. The pituitary gland, not the ovaries, governs the production of milk. By applying the right techniques, most women can produce at least some.

Adoptive mothers can now receive help from lactation consultants, adoption agencies, and websites on how to induce lactation so they can breastfeed their babies. Although the majority of women who have tried this to date haven't been able produce enough milk for all their baby's needs, it is believed that even a few drops of breastmilk will make a difference to its health, and to the quality of the parent-child relationship.

In the 1980s a pair of Australian sisters, Maggie and Linda Kirkman, became famous for successfully performing the first surrogate pregnancy. The younger sister, Linda Kirkman, agreed that she would bear her sister's child, using Maggie's ovum and an anonymous donor's sperm, but only on the condition that once born, Maggie would breastfeed her own child. Their best-selling book, *My Sister's Child*, includes the story of Maggie's success.

The health benefits to women of lactating also make the effort worthwhile. A ten-year study by Cancer Research UK, whose results were published in *The Lancet* in July 2002, concluded that women can significantly reduce their risk of breast cancer by breastfeeding as long as possible. The relative risk of breast cancer was found to decrease by 4.3 percent for every twelve months of breastfeeding, in addition to a decrease of 7 percent for each birth. Helen Studd of the *London Times* reported, "If British women were to have more children, who are breastfed for two years each, the disease would be all but wiped out."

The knowledge that women can induce lactation without having any children at all makes this information even more explosive. What if women were to lactate simply for their own good health? What other reasons would be needed to justify lactating for partners, or for the purpose of trying out a larger breast size, or just for the hell of it? The possibilities of recreational lactation open up a vista of opportunities for pleasure, not to mention an excuse to shop for new bras and other gadgets. A range of sleek breast pumps designed by

Philippe Starck cannot be far away, especially as it's already been reported, in the *New York Times*, that a "pumping vest" is on the market, allowing a woman to go about her business while the vest supposedly works discreetly.

Sandra Steingraber's work for the Cornell Program on Breast Cancer and Environmental Risk Factors has also argued strongly for the health benefits of lactating as a means of ridding women's bodies of toxins. She writes, "The problem with dioxins, and other fat-soluble persistent contaminants, is that you can't easily metabolize and pee them out. Lactation, which does remove fat from a woman's body, is the only effective way to purge dioxin from the body." The results are impressive. A Swedish study concluded that one American women who breastfed her twins for three years "dropped her body burden of dioxins by 69 percent."

This of course raises fears in mothers' minds that they are passing toxins on to their babies when they breastfeed, an anxiety that the tabloid press has been quick to exploit. However, Steingraber counsels that breastmilk is still superior to formula as a food for children. This is partly because formula is so deficient biochemically, and partly because the extra body fat put on during pregnancy specifically to fuel milk production is new, and therefore is virtually toxin-free. It is only in the stored fat, where a lifetime of pollutants might have built up, that problems lie, especially for older mothers who were exposed to higher levels of DDT and dioxins. If it were better known that women could lactate before giving birth, they could rid their bodies of any possible contamination whenever they pleased, benefiting both themselves and their babies. (Women who have HIV-AIDS or hepatitis C, however, should consult the latest information before breast-feeding, as HIV can be transmitted through breatsmilk, and hepatitis C via blood from cracked nipples.)

Older women who missed out on breastfeeding when having their own children could also benefit—by inducing lactation either for their health or for their grandchildren. In the following story, there is an anecdote about a grandmother who confesses to surreptitiously breastfeeding her grand-child. While I was researching this book, an Australian woman told me how her own mother, now living in Bali, began lactating when baby-sitting her first grandchild, and subsequently helped out. Given the large number of grand-mothers who have never had the opportunity to breastfeed and might now regret this, it is tempting to wonder if induc-ing lactation would be both helpful to their daughters and healing to themselves.

In the meantime, it is the adoptive and surrogate mothers who are leading the way, showing how, once given the right support and advice, breastfeeding is possible for virtually all women. Like any fitness program, all you need is an enthusi-asm for pumping, and commitment.

~ ⌐

My husband and I learned in November 1997 that we were going to be having Elizabeth in January. We went to San Antonio to meet the birth mother at Thanksgiving. At about the same time, I became acquainted with two women in Austin, Cindy and Naomi, who had successfully breastfed their adopted children. They became a support group for me. Cindy was still nursing her biological daughter as well as her nine-month-old adopted son. Naomi had nursed her adopted daughter until she was about two years old. These women were wonderful contacts for the experiences they had gone through in inducing lactation. I also sought the advice of a lactation consultant, Barbara Wilson-Clay. I will always remember how she joked that telephone support was available to me until my child turned eighteen. Barbara was my lifeline. I also networked and talked to many different people and was reading as much as I could.

I started using a breast pump on January 1, and Elizabeth was due on the twenty-first, so I thought I had twenty-one days to prepare my breasts to feed our daughter. I was pumping about four times a day for about twenty minutes each side. Over the first few days I pumped, I was not certain my breasts were changing all that much. I do remember that they started to seem larger, and there were unquestionably some hormonal changes taking place in my body. Within days I had started to produce a few drops of chocolate-colored milk. It was very motivating to have something happening so quickly!

I asked Barbara why my milk had this color. She assured me that this was fine, that we do not have much information about the range of color of initial mother's milk because it is generally ingested. With time, my expressed milk became more traditional in color.

Part of my preparation for nursing included making changes to my diet. These changes had started years earlier, while I was being treated for endometriosis and infertility. The most dramatic change I made was to follow a rotation diet, where I avoided wheat and rotated the grains I ate each day on a schedule of every two to four days (depending on the type of grain and how the body tolerates it).

I also tried some homeopathic treatments, which seemed to help me get my allergy symptoms under control.

A doctor I spoke to advised me that nonpasteurized, nonalcoholic beer is useful for supporting milk production. Evidently the hops are excellent for encouraging a good supply of milk. I found two brands of German nonalcoholic beer at our neighborhood market and both were very good—Haake Beck and Clausthaler. I would drink one or two bottles each day. I also took two fenugreek tablets three times a day with meals, and drank Mother's Milk Tea, which contains fennel, anise, coriander, and fenugreek seed as well as spearmint leaf, lemongrass, lemon verbena leaf, althea root, and blessed thistle leaf. I was advised to arrange for lots of nurturing massage—of tummy, throat, and breasts—and to use visualization of the baby at the breast when I pumped, to help with the release of prolactin, the hormone that stimulates milk production. I also underwent treatment by an acupuncturist for several weeks to help bring in my milk supply and increase production.

I work as a lecturer at a university, so I was on teaching break during the first part of January. I had hoped to get everything organized, as well as the baby on track, before I was due back to teach. I was counting on those twenty-one days to get things in order in the house and to get my milk supply established. Unfortunately, we were not able to achieve these goals. On the twelfth of January Elizabeth decided she was ready to come meet her mommy and daddy. I am so thankful I was already producing some milk!

My husband and I had talked to the birth mother the evening before and she seemed on schedule, but on Monday morning, January twelfth, the birth mom called to let us know she had gone into labor.

Within thirty minutes we had gathered everything we needed

and asked various neighbors and friends to take care of mail, newspaper, rented videos, and such tasks; and there was an accident a few blocks from home that slowed us down even more. My husband commented that it was a good thing I'd made a list of everything we should have with us, since we were not thinking too clearly as we packed the car.

The drive from Austin to San Antonio takes about one-and-a-half hours. As we drove, I prepared our backpack with the items we wanted to take with us into the hospital. I also moved into the backseat to pump for a few minutes as we traveled. The trip went smoothly, and we arrived at the hospital shortly after the birth mom did.

The birth mother had agreed that I should be present at the birth, and so I coached her, giving her ice, massage, and wet compresses as she would accept them through the painful contractions. It was very intense and she clearly experienced a great deal of pain; in spite of that, she smiled a bit from time to time at things the doctor, nurse, or I said to her. I was holding her hand when our baby, Miss Elizabeth, entered into the world at 2:00 P.M. It was very exciting. She was just a very sweet purple baby.

This was not our birth mother's first child, and she had made clear to both the doctor and the hospital staff that this baby was not destined to be hers. She was fully committed to us as this child's parents. The doctor and nurses were wonderfully supportive.

My husband and I were warmly welcomed into the hospital nursery as Elizabeth was measured, cleaned, and checked. The nurses encouraged me to try to nurse her. I was prepared to use a lactation aid called an SNS (Supplemental Nursing System), which consists of a small hard plastic bottle suspended around the mother's neck, with two tiny tubes running from the bottle cap at the bottom of the bottle. The tubing is taped in place against the breast to position it properly at the nipple. This allows the baby to latch on and nurse, with the only difference from "regular" nursing being the small tube she takes into her mouth with the nipple. The baby receives as much milk from the SNS bottle as she needs to supplement what is coming from the mother's breast. For a mother without an adequate milk supply, as in my case, the lactation aid is a vital backup to ensure proper nutrition.

My first few attempts to feed Elizabeth in the nursery were not successful. We had difficulties getting her to latch on correctly; the setting was not very private; she was quite sleepy; and we were all somewhat unfamiliar with the process. Policy dictated that she must ingest something before she would be allowed to leave the nursery, so the nurse offered us several options for how to deliver her first meal. We did not want to use a bottle, since we were concerned that this would confuse Elizabeth. The nurse suggested a gravity-fed tube to her stomach, which would not require her to suckle. So that is how she got her first meal. The process went very quickly; and now it was time to move Elizabeth into her birth mother's room.

My husband spent the night with friends while I roomed in with Elizabeth and the birth mother. Every time the baby became hungry during the night, I tried nursing her again. The room was quite dark, and I was in an uncomfortable chair designed to pull out to a narrow bed. Elizabeth had a hard time finding what she was looking for but we kept trying. She was so sleepy that it was difficult to stick with it long enough to succeed. In the light of morning we discovered that I had little baby hickey marks all over my breasts!

The next day, Wednesday, was a long one; the doctor did not come to OK the release until nine o'clock at night. The birth mother and baby were finally released from the hospital two hours later, at eleven o'clock on January 13. We drove the birth mother home and then took our baby with us, at long last, to the hotel room where we would stay until the placement was completed. The privacy and comfort of our room helped all of us relax and become acquainted. As soon as we settled in that night, I fed Elizabeth and continued to feed her on demand. My husband and I monitored her intake as well as how frequently she was producing wet or soiled diapers. We basically camped out on the big king-sized bed in our room and focused on Elizabeth's moment-to-moment needs.

Part of the challenge with getting in sync with feeding was that it was all new to me, as it is for any first-time mother. The lactation consultant from the hospital conferred with me in person and by phone, which helped me work through some discouraging episodes. The birth mom was supportive too. She chose not to feed Elizabeth at all and left it entirely to me. She took medication to dry up her own milk supply as quickly as possible. I think she found it was rather novel that I was so interested in breastfeeding Elizabeth.

One of the more interesting things about my case is that I am post-menopausal. I went through a lot of infertility treatments in the early 1990s. In 1993 I was diagnosed with endometriosis. My treatment for this included four months of treatment with Lupron, a hormone that induced pseudomenopause in order to shrink the endometrial growths. I had major surgery in May of 1993, followed by continued hormone treatments. A year later the specialist mentioned offhandedly, "Well, I guess you just have early ovarian shutdown."

His statement angered me and made me feel that I needed to take matters into my own hands. In retrospect, I was unhappy about some of the choices that I was led to, as well as the attitudes, which seemed focused on the technical challenges of causing my body to do what others wanted it to do. The process had certainly not considered the influence that any other aspects of my health and well-being might have had on my fertility.

I decided that day to stop following the mainstream medical route and embarked on a more natural dietary and herbal approach to my problems. I was still hopeful that it would not be "too late," since I had read various stories of miraculous results in conception. But my gynecologist did the hormonal tests to check my status and confirmed that I was well into menopause at the age of forty.

After my husband and I decided to become parents via adoption, I was still committed to breastfeeding our baby, but I was concerned that being postmenopausal would make it harder for me to lactate. This was something I had researched a bit when we started considering adoption. I remember talking to Barbara, my lactation consultant, about grandmothers who breastfed, so I knew postmenopausal lactation was possible. In part I was hopeful that my body could still contribute to our daughter's sustenance. I also knew that establishing a breastfeeding relationship was a key part of the way I wanted to mother my child.

So here I was, more than two years after being told I was menopausal, producing milk and noticing clear hormonal changes occurring in my body. My breasts had atrophied after the endometriosis treatments, but as I induced lactation they quickly became fuller, even larger than they were before menopause. Three years of breastfeeding later, they are still quite filled out.

It was very exciting when I started experiencing letdown after Elizabeth was several months old. I thought, "Oh! Things are moving!" It literally felt like the milk was moving. I found it almost painful, as if the milk molecules were wider than the ducts they passed through, and it caused a tingling sensation. It was like a very strong movement in the breasts, like a message of greeting and renewal coming from my body. I still love the feeling of letdown. I feel it confirms my contributions to her nutrition.

When Elizabeth was three months old, I discovered a different kind of lactation aid, called a Lactaid, which uses a soft bag instead of a hard plastic bottle but also lies against the chest. I found it was much more comfortable to wear, in part because it conformed to the contours of my body. Even better, the single tube from the Lactaid device could be positioned against my nipple without the need for tape. That was one of the things that sold me on it. No tape—what a lovely thought! The bag hangs around the mother's neck and can be adjusted for height—I always let the bag hang as low as possible. The tube winds over and across the breast. I usually curve it up toward the nipple so it extends just past the end of the nipple. Then I support the breast with my hand, holding the tube with my thumb, while I use the other hand to guide the baby to latch on. When it is time to switch sides, I simply switch the process to the other hand. The tiny feeding tube on the Lactaid is much softer than the pair on the SNS, which I believe is the reason the tape-free approach works so well.

Losing the tape and the hard bottle converted me in one use; I have never looked back. Some mothers have told me they prefer the SNS; they complained that the soft bag is harder to fill and tips over more easily. My husband and I have not had problems with this; we keep six devices on hand so we can fill enough for several feedings at once. In Austin, the Lactaid equipment is not available in a store, so we order what we need via telephone and the Internet. It has worked out very well. I have to tell you, it was so nice to stop putting tape on my breasts. The tape caused terrible irritation, even when I used the most skin-sensitive tape. Gravity is also less of a factor with the Lactaid than with the SNS. This means the mother can be in any position to feed, even lying down. While I did lie down sometimes with the

SNS, we had to be more creative with where to position it in order to ensure a constant flow of milk.

An interesting note about the SNS is that it comes with three sets of feeding tubes in different sizes. We started feeding Elizabeth using one of the smallest set of tubes; but when Elizabeth was about two-and-a-half weeks old, our lactation consultant suggested that the small size of the tubes was forcing Elizabeth to work too hard to get enough formula. We switched to the larger tubes, and Elizabeth's feeding sessions became much more productive; she did not become tired as quickly. When we switched to the Lactaid device, tube size was not an issue. That device comes with only one tube size, and the rate of delivery is determined exclusively by the child's rate of intake.

Early on I had my one horrible day. I ended up calling the La Leche League. The night before, my nipples had become too sensitive, so I was finger-feeding Elizabeth using the SNS (a technique that my husband could also use). In the middle of the night, when I was very exhausted, Elizabeth actually ingested the tape I had used to attach the SNS tube to my finger. When I took my finger away from her mouth, the tape was gone! I felt like the most terrible mother in the world. It evolved into a crisis day where everything led to tears.

I had returned to teaching when Elizabeth was only nine days old. Much of the stress was from suddenly being a parent, especially a working parent, and I had to figure it all out. I was teaching three mornings a week. During the time I was in the classroom and at office hours (about four hours), my husband stayed at home with Elizabeth. He would feed her with a bottle or with his finger using the lactation device. Elizabeth did well during these times, although she was always very happy to be put back to the breast when I came home again. I feel that these regular opportunities for them to be together without having me around as immediate backup allowed them to build a very close bond. We never felt that Elizabeth became confused at the variety of approaches to feeding; she seemed to settle into the attitude that the bottle was how Daddy fed her, while the breast was how Mommy fed her.

There is a wide range of possible milk production in adoptive mothers, just as there is in birth mothers. The age of the woman, her hormonal status, the reason for her infertility—all these factors can influence the potential milk supply. For me, the reward is the experience of breastfeeding and the enhanced bonding from the skin-to-skin contact. Any amount of milk my body makes is a welcome bonus.

Barbara, my lactation consultant, shared several articles with me before Elizabeth arrived. One, from the *Journal of Tropical Pediatrics,* was a study in Papua New Guinea of some women who had induced lactation when adopting a child. Most of the women in that study developed a full milk supply. However, they tended to be young women who were adopting babies from family members who had been killed or who could not cope. This means that these women probably represent a different population than most Western women, who are most likely to be inducing lactation when they are older. Barbara tells me that she has worked with lots of adoptive moms and has never personally seen such a woman make a full milk supply. Some of her clients have made as much as twenty ounces a day, but many seem to make as little as two to four ounces a day. There is clearly a wide range of possibilities, which depend on each woman's physiology.

I knew from the start that it was very unlikely that I would be able to develop a sufficient supply of milk quickly enough to sustain

Elizabeth on my breastmilk alone. Before she arrived, my husband and I had talked about what we would do if I was unable to induce lactation. We agreed that while producing breastmilk would be nice, it was not the main point.

In retrospect, I think that even if Elizabeth had waited the additional nine days to arrive, I still would not have been producing enough breastmilk. Even months later, I was uncertain how much I was contributing to her intake. One day when she was several months old, I had her with me at my university office. While I was nursing her, I happened to look down at the other breast and think, Well, I wonder if I can express milk? I tried it, and it worked! It was very exciting and somewhat surprising. I had never needed to learn how to express properly, so my technique was not very good!

Expressing the milk was a great reconfirmation. I had come to feel a little bit like an imposter, thinking, "I am putting my baby to my breast, but that is all, her nutrition is just what is in this bag." It was thrilling when I could express some milk and see, "Oh, something is going on here!" I still check every once in a while and confirm that I am still producing milk.

A year or so back, I was traveling with Elizabeth and spoke to an older woman at the airport. We connected because she was carrying a child in a rebozo, a type of traditional Mexican shawl that I also used for babywearing. We talked about how lovely it is to use the rebozo. This woman turned out to be the child's grandmother. It was clear that she was something of an earth mother. This was in strong contrast to her daughter who, she told me, was very conservative and had weaned the baby early. The grandmother admitted to me that she had put the baby to her own breast a few times.

Elizabeth is now three and a half years old and I am still nursing her three times a day. She has developed her own terminology to let me know whether she wants to feed with the bag or without. A "little bite" means nursing without the bag, and a "big bite" means she would like to feed with the Lactaid. The little bite is more or less to touch base with Mom and have some physical contact. I know that sometimes when she needs a little bite, it is because my schedule has become too demanding. The nursing helps guarantee that we sit down together. I know that is part of why nursing feels important for us: at those times I put aside everything else and I am with her completely.

I knew from the beginning that I would continue breastfeeding Elizabeth for the long haul. I see no reason to wean Elizabeth until she is clearly ready to stop. I feel that yielding to pressure from the outside is the wrong reason to stop. I cannot imagine parenting without the breastfeeding component. I know intellectually that it is possible, but I do not understand the choice not to breastfeed. I was not breastfed when I was born. It just was something that people did not do, so my mother was discouraged from doing it. By the time my sister was born four years later, she was breastfed, as was my brother, who was born another six years after that. I have often wondered whether not being breastfed influenced my tendency to have allergies, or other aspects of my health. My mother is no longer here to ask questions about these things, or about parenting, or to better understand how my siblings and I were raised.

A year ago, our family was thrilled at the opportunity to become part of the support network for our neighbors, who adopted a child when Elizabeth was about two and a half years old. They tried to induce lactation, but found that this did not work for their family for a variety of reasons. It is touching, though, that the first baby who has become a regular part of Elizabeth's life came to his family in the same way that Elizabeth came to ours.

It's also wonderful that we have a continuing relationship with Elizabeth's birth mother. We get together around Elizabeth's birthday every year. She is still too young to understand the meaning her birth mother has in her life, but we hope that their ongoing relationship will help her make sense of her place in the world.

Tran

The following story evolved after a young mother emailed me to confess that she was sexually aroused during breastfeeding. She was anxious to know if this was common, and wanted to find out more about it. I reassured her that she wasn't alone, and passed on to her some of the erotic fiction about lactation that I had come across. In the process she told me her story, a candid and joyful account of her polymorphous sex life and fantasies.

At the same time, I was receiving questionnaire answers that indicated more than a few women were either sexually aroused while breastfeeding, or wished they had been relaxed enough at the time to explore this possibility. One woman pointed out: "As to my husband and my sex life, it was transformed by breastfeeding. When the milk came down at the beginning of a feed it was like the beginning of an orgasm (in fact my sex life took off after being able to have an orgasm more easily), so I felt like having sex while breastfeeding, and we did. My husband and I both realized that it was good for foreplay, and this has fortunately continued after our babies have grown up. . . . I cannot understand other people's reaction to feeding. For me and for my husband it was a decided turn-on. He enjoyed sucking on my lactating breasts as my baby did. What a bonus!"

Another woman wrote that since weaning her child, her breasts had become "more sensitive, more erotic. . . . Before babies, sexual play involving my breasts did very little to excite me. Now they are a major erogenous zone."

Many women find that becoming a mother does not always sit easily with the sexual identity they formed before becoming pregnant. We are instructed to wait for six weeks after delivery to have sex, but it often takes much longer to rework the fantasies and rebuild a picture of ourselves as sexual individuals. As Margaret Christakos writes in her poem "Bits," in which a nursing mother addresses her child:

> *Holding ourselves back is de rigueur*
> *your mouth on my breast could bite as easily*
> *& I could swell with erotic desire*
>
> *or vanish, instead*

For many new mothers, allowing their body to vanish from their erotic imagination seems the easiest solution, not only while breastfeeding, but for some time afterward. For others, becoming invisible just isn't an option, as the sexual responsiveness of their breasts while lactating results in floods of milk, impossible to conceal. One woman spoke for many others when she wrote, "My breasts would often start shooting milk when I came."

For some this was a turn-on, for others a nuisance. As

Adrienne Rich points out in *Of Woman Born,* "The act of suckling a child, like a sexual act, may be tense, physically painful, charged with cultural feelings of inadequacy and guilt. Or, like a sexual act, it can be a physically delicious, elementally soothing experience, filled with a tender sensuality."

One respondent stated, "I despise nipple stimulation, and find it very irritating except [in] exceptional circumstances." Another scaled new heights of pleasure: "With each baby my breasts became more and more sensitive and erogenous. During the last pregnancy it was absolutely mind-blowing how erotic they were to the touch. . . . I think the idea of breastfeeding again made me connect to my feelings as a 'woman and earth mother' in a very erotic sense. My partner responded to this admirably."

The postpartum body not only looks different, but may be traumatized, at least temporarily. And for many women, it seems to have fulfilled its function as a sexual turn-on, becoming instead a strictly utilitarian zone deployed for feeding, cuddling, and carrying—and if you've produced budding athletes, sometimes as a trampoline. Many a father too is taken aback by the experience of watching his partner give birth, and sometimes needs time before he can think of her again as sexually desirable.

In one of the most touching replies I received, a woman wrote that she had been under a serious misapprehension about the lack of appeal her postlactating breasts held for her husband. She wrote: "I had to tell you about feeling my breasts are ugly since becoming a mom six years ago, and keeping them covered from my husband. Then I found the bottom bit [of the questionnaire] was for men, so yesterday evening I ran through it with my husband, and was shocked shocked shocked to find that he doesn't consider my breasts ugly at all, and in fact thinks of them in a somewhat sexier way now than in their 'virginal' state! It was a totally huge thing for me to find out and has opened up an aspect of our relationship I'd closed off ages ago."

As one male respondent, who stated that "I love my partner's breasts even more," went on to say: "The whole process of raising a child changes the way you relate sexually. . . . I always related to my wife as a very sexy woman. Breastfeeding didn't really change that feeling much. . . . I didn't have any fantasies about breastfeeding, but I suppose I was attracted to her added 'maternalness.' . . . I am just turned on by my wife in any form or shape she happens to be in."

Apart from qualifying as the perfect husband, this man points out the futility of attempts, whether by men or women, to separate the various roles a woman's body is called on to perform. As one woman succinctly put it, "Sometimes during foreplay or when I had orgasms I would spontaneously lactate anyway, so it didn't really matter that I wanted to keep everything all nice and tidy. My body had its way, as it always does."

From my own experience, I know that my old sexual fantasies, many of them dating back to adolescence, simply didn't work anymore. Some of them even made me laugh. In the meantime, waiting for new and more enticing perspectives to emerge, it sometimes seemed easier to split off the new maternal identity from the old sexual one, and shut down the libido until it was possible to integrate the two selves into some fabulously well-adjusted domestic goddess. Little wonder that for many women and men, the lactating breast—

engorged, radiating heat, its nipples darkened and erect—provides a bridge to a renewed sex life.

But this can take time, both in adjusting to motherhood and in adapting to long-term breastfeeding, which then allows for ovulation to reestablish itself, and for the hormones that fire up libido to kick in. As one woman wrote:

> I wasn't going to be celibate for eighteen months (which turned out to be the median age I fed all three children). My boobs were a no-go zone for the most part. . . . I didn't like letting down and getting milk everywhere. This wasn't that much of a hardship—you adjust. As I was weaning the third child, my second partner was given unprecedented access to my breasts—I was extraordinarily turned on at that time by the fact that he was getting milk when he sucked on them. Call me weird. Three babies down the track and I have developed an erotic association with myself as a nurturer—even to my lover. I love my breasts, they've done a wonderful job, and continue to amaze and delight me with their responsiveness to stimuli. I never confused the connection, though. Apart from a handful of isolated instances when I got horny from feeding my babies, I never associated them as an erogenous zone while feeding. I just became increasingly sensitive over time to breast stimulation in the bedroom.

For some women, it is not maternal weariness, or an uncertain sexual identity, but the fear of being accused of incest that has made them reticent about acknowledging or exploring anything but the most subtle of pleasures when engaging with their babies. Maternal virtue and nutritional excellence—not pleasure—is what we've been taught breast-feeding is supposed to promote.

According to Noel Oxenhandler, author of *The Eros of Parenthood*, it is precisely this overheated anxiety about parent-child intimacy that increases the risk of incest. With the narrowing of sexual definitions to account only for inter-course, there is a loss of knowledge to understand, and vocabulary to describe, the many other sexual behaviors and urges of the human animal, including children. Nonorgasmic but nevertheless intensely sensual forms of embodied con-nection are at the heart of loving parent-child attachment, and part of the spectrum of affectionate exchange between individuals generally. Because breastfeeding encompasses both erotic and maternal physiology, it has unfortunately been policed by overzealous child welfare workers, leading in some cases to state-enforced weaning.

In 2000 a woman in Champaign, Illinois, was separated from her five-year-old son for nine months after being reported by her baby-sitter for breastfeeding. Even more startling, in 1991 a young mother in Syracuse, New York, was taken into custody and separated from her baby daughter for a year after calling a help line to get advice on mild feelings of sexual arousal that she'd experienced while breastfeeding. In Australia in 1998 the Family Court ordered a nursing mother to wean her fourteen-month-old son so that his father could have overnight access. The court stated that "the mother could . . . cause psychological harm" by continuing to nurse beyond this age, and drew from a psychiatrist's report concluding that "prolonged breastfeeding might be a sign of the mother's emotional problems."

Asked to comment on the Illinois case, Oxenhandler told the *New York Times,* "We were in denial about the reality of child abuse for so long that it's understandable that we have reacted with a black and white mentality. I think it's time to find a middle ground where we can acknowledge that the erotic pleasure that propels us to reproduce is part of the same pleasure that propels us to nurture our children, and that's something to be celebrated, not denied. It's a truism of psychology that what we can't acknowledge is what causes problems."

As the lactation consultant and author Barbara Wilson-Clay once told me, "I believe breastfeeding can work as a biological protection against child abuse."

Most parents of small children will at some stage weather the problem of finding the time and energy for sexual intimacy and exploring the altered landscape of their relationship. The incorporation of breastfeeding into their sexual lives, the relaxing of the divisions between the mother's maternal and sexual identity, together with an encouragement to fathers to engage in close physical affection with their children, might not only help to make breastfeeding possible over longer periods, but also aid in maintaining harmony between all the family members.

As Margaret Christakos continues, in her poem, to muse on her baby at her breast:

You coax me toward the common interest
the human problem of growing up
gradually
drag me by one nipple to a reckoning
with how sexy we are

soft breast your eye is up against constantly
eunuch skin of your cheek, bellows I adore
in a cycle of puffing, sucking
chuffing like a pony's nostril as it labours
around the demands of a premature bridle
this new & more appropriate morality
where my tit is a temple now
around which we gather and gaze and supplicate

The suspense of feeling
is killing me sometimes I think
I will forget where I'm leading you, lapse

& feel it
& have to pull you off quickly
away from who I've been in the world up till now
before I installed my heart in my mouth
& came here like a virgin
to serve you

I remember a friend telling me she went to this all-night party and her breasts got really hard so her partner emptied them for her by sucking all the milk out. I think that would really turn me on. I would love a partner who was really into the erotic nature of breastmilk. It would make me feel honored as a woman and as a mother—kind of like a goddess!

—Reply to questionnaire

*B*oth my pregnancies were A-one! I felt wonderful, and sex was better than before, mostly because for the first time ever, I had a woman's figure. I'd never really thought how self-conscious I was about my flat chest before my boobs started to swell.

I have long nipples. My cousin and best friend always said, from when I was about thirteen, "You mightn't have any boobs but your nipples have sure popped." And since then she always just says, "Pop!" to me, as a kind of shorthand joke between us.

And I always got heaps of response to nipple stimulation right from the time when they first grew. But now my husband can suck on *boobs* as well. Actually, he could suck them totally into his mouth, and still can, and I love that.

Plus I think there has been heaps more blood flow round the pubic area ever since I fell pregnant. Let's be frank, my lips and clit have swelled enormously. It's really obvious when they are black, and you're bald, because my pubic hair never grew—not that this is unusual in Chinese, I think.

Not that I really know. I'd virtually never seen anyone naked before I came to Australia. It was a total eye-opener, going to boarding school. Communal showers! Virtually all the non-Asian girls, and even a few of us, too, walked around topless, and quite a few didn't seem to care if you saw them naked, even outside the showers. It took me a while to get used to that! It was really important to me to fit in (and still is, if I'm totally honest). And then I eventually realized I was actually less conspicuous if I did as the Romans did. To tell the truth, I got quite a kick out of seeing and being seen. In some ways my sexuality was formed then. Now it totally blows me away being watched masturbating. My heart pumps like it is about to burst and my chest gets so tight, I feel I can hardly breathe. I now know how Victorian ladies in novels must have felt when they swooned.

I always felt that breastfeeding would be best for my babies, and when I discovered how much I liked it, which was a lot, that was a big bonus. I had some slight soreness from breastfeeding at first but nothing really serious, and no problems at all once I got started. I was sort of shocked, though, at how wet I got "down there." (That's my mother's expression—gross, hey?)

From pretty much the first time I started breastfeeding I would become aroused. Now I think it's almost a reflex. But I was shocked at first, when I realized what was happening, and decided to ignore it. Then I realized that's nuts, so now I let it build up, and then rub myself when the baby's finished feeding.

Having such responsive breasts helped me overcome any hesitation either my husband or I may have felt about having sex again after I gave birth—touching my breasts got us both horny so quickly. Then, one night in bed, my husband said he'd like to try my milk, and started sucking. I was a bit shocked, to tell the truth, but my milk just flowed in about five seconds flat! He also fingered me as he sucked, and I came straight away. My orgasms are always stronger after he's been breastfeeding.

We talked about it too. He likes feeding from me, but he also likes me expressing over his face and his cock. There, I've said it—my mother would die!

I've also incorporated my new breasts into masturbation. I'd always sort of rolled my nipples with one hand while rubbing the hood of my clit with the other, and I just kept on doing it. I sort of milk my clit through the hood, something I've always done if I have plenty of time. Now that I'm lactating, the milk starts to come out of my breasts, so there's always milk everywhere, and I have to lie on a thick towel.

Sometimes I wake in the morning to find my husband is nursing from me. He just sucks, the milk starts, and the letdown wakes me up, and we start bonking, or he rubs his penis against me and I masturbate, or he finger-fucks me.

I've also fallen asleep with him feeding on me, many times. My husband seems to fall asleep sometimes too, though if I reach down, he's still hard.

I've still been feeding my second baby while we're doing this, although not at the same time that my husband nurses. She sometimes shares the bed, but is most often in her cot. I'm not comfortable having sex while breastfeeding. My mother on my shoulder again!

My five-year-old, who I weaned at three, is very matter-of-fact about my breasts, and doesn't take much notice of my body, though about six months ago he hurt himself and was very upset, and was happy to feed for a day or so.

I did worry at first that my husband might be taking all my milk, and there'd not be enough for my baby, but it wasn't a problem at all. In fact, when he was away for a week or ten days with work, the supply slowed, but as soon as he came back it increased again. I've always had too much milk, really, and I always hand-express when I shower. So my husband's involvement is good for helping me to regulate my supply in a way, and my milk seems to adjust very quickly to demand.

I've decided I'm going to continue lactating for as long as possible, just for the sex. My husband kept feeding after the first one was pretty much weaned, and he certainly doesn't intend to let me dry out after this one finishes. And that's more than fine by me!

Breastfeeding in public is a different matter. I don't feel relaxed at all. No way. For all my liberated pretensions, I can still feel the disapproval of my mother and her cronies if I even *think* about doing it.

But with my girlfriend it's the opposite, and I *really* like them seeing my boobs. I also have sexual fantasies about other women seeing me express. When I was at school, I saw one of my school friend's moms expressing when I stayed on their property, and couldn't believe it. We burst into her dressing room without warning and she was expressing into the basin. She wasn't at all fussed, nor was my friend, who said she did that because her boobies were too swollen for her baby to feed. I was amazed she was letting me see that, and I was also amazed at how much milk she produced, and how far the jets of milk shot out.

The other thing I'd *really* like is for each of my two best friends to feed on me, and it's almost happened with each of them—I'm hopeful it won't be too long as I'm sure they're both interested. I've been wanting to set it up so they'll ask, because otherwise it won't happen—I'm too afraid of rejection. But what I'd like is for them to just sort of hint, and then I'd let them, and we'd each masturbate slowly for the rest of the afternoon.

I Did It!

The idea of cooking with breastmilk is, to many, peculiar if not repulsive. Natalie Angier writes in her book *Woman: An Intimate Geography*, "If you saw a full glass of human milk in the refrigerator, would you drink it? The idea is disturbing. It feels almost cannibalistic."

Breast milk is a bodily fluid, and we have been taught that, as such, it should be treated with care, especially if there is a risk of infection. Although the risk of being infected by breastmilk is negligible, the fact that it is stuff that comes out of our bodies means that it's associated with everything from urine to blood, sweat, and saliva. It makes perfect sense that some of these fluids are strictly regulated. It has often been remarked, after all, that the efficiently flushing toilet is the one truly great contribution, along with jazz, made by America to Western civilization.

But breastmilk seems to have been unnecessarily caught up in a swirl of squeamishness. It's not just a bodily fluid, after all. It's also a food. The fact that it comes out of a woman's bosom, and not a cow's udder, shouldn't reduce its appeal, from a rational point of view, and might increase it when considering its compatibility to the needs of the human body. As one mother wrote, "One day I had some breastmilk in the fridge and my girlfriend went to put it in her tea. When I told her what it was she freaked. But it is incongruous because what you are basically saying is that you would rather have milk from some old fly-ridden cow in a muddy field than from your best friend. Seems rather strange."

Several other women who answered the questionnaire confessed to putting breastmilk in tea, or using it in cooking, or on breakfast cereal. "I tricked a doctor once and put it in his tea. He never knew," wrote one lactation consultant with obvious relish. Another wrote, more apologetically, "My mom once put some expressed breastmilk into her minister's tea when he called and she didn't have any [cows'] milk and was so embarrassed that in desperation she used her own. He said it was the nicest cup of tea he'd ever had!"

Another commented matter-of-factly, "I once was making a pie, and the recipe called for the crust to be brushed with milk, then sprinkled with sugar. I was out of cows' milk, so I just expressed some milk over the crust and added the sugar. I have used it in other recipes too. Nobody ever notices."

There is another bodily fluid that is also regulated, like breastmilk, for no apparent reason. This fluid is tears. Similarly untainted by any real risk of infection, it is nevertheless a substance that can cause consternation if allowed to flow freely in public. Perhaps it has to do with maintaining a clear boundary between infant and adult behavior. Children may cry in public, but adults should not, unless excused by extreme circumstances. Similarly, small children may breast-feed, but older ones should not, lest this should cause offense to onlookers, or suggest that a child's needs may run rampant across its mother's body, and at the expense of its father's desire. This is especially true among those who see parenting and sex as mutually exclusive.

Many writers have noted the connection between tears and breastmilk, and some have described nipples as eyes. This is not simply because breastfeeding mothers may be seen to weep. Both milk and tears are expressed. They are a substance that communicates an affect—from pain and sadness to love and longing—and can be stimulated by the sight of a loved one. Their relationship to the nervous system is unique. It is not necessary to expel their fluid on a regular basis, but only under certain conditions. And sometimes they resist expression at all. Just as stress can inhibit letdown, so can shock, or depression, inhibit tears. And the appearance of either has been known, throughout history, to quicken a lover's heart.

Breastmilk is also used medicinally, in the treatment of patients with severe allergies and immune disorders. Many mothers are taught that its sterile properties make it perfect for curing conjunctivitis in babies, or healing cracked nipples or excema. One lactation consultant told me how her neighbor's children would line up to receive a squirt of her breastmilk in their eyes, at times when pinkeye took hold in their suburb. Another mother wrote that she would give breastmilk to her older, weaned children "when they were feeling ill." Another woman wrote, "I gave my husband breastmilk to drink for a few months while he was undergoing chemotherapy for lupus. He said that he only liked to drink it fresh and warm; not from the fridge. We told his rheumatologist about the breastmilk and he was a little surprised, but said go for it. . . . If I had an intestinal bug again and was still lactating, I would drink [my] breastmilk."

The medicinal use of breastmilk is centuries old, and has only recently been rediscovered by contemporary medicine, particularly in the treatment of immunodeficiency disorders. The historian Marylynn Salmon writes of the case of the Reverend Ebenezer Parkman, who lay on his deathbed in Boston in 1752. She quotes from his diary of August 21: "I am so wasted, that there appears to me Danger of consuming away." After he suffered several more days of fever and rheumatic pain, his wife, Hannah, sent her one-year-old baby, Samuel, off for weaning and breastfed her husband instead. Parkman records the event in his journal: "My wife tends me o'nights and supply's me with Breast: milky." As Salmon writes, "Little Samuel's loss was Ebenezer's gain. The father recovered from his illness to live another thirty years."

Salmon's article goes on to document the many remedies based on breastmilk in sixteenth-century literature, showing how it was prescribed for pain relief, eye infections, consumption, and liver disorders, among other ailments. She writes, "As late as the second half of the eighteenth century, breast milk still was recommended as an ingredient in medicinal recipes."

One questionnaire respondent, apparently a reader of historical novels, wrote: "I have also read stories of men in the Middle Ages who couldn't eat after a vicious sword wound to the stomach and would surely die because of this, as well as infection, yet taking breastmilk from their nursing wives, [they] slowly gained their health without taxing their stomachs with heavier foods." She went on to note, "Maybe if

we drank breastmilk instead of cows' milk there would be
fewer allergies and less obesity in this world. Breastmilk is
very easily digested, so I imagine people who suffer bowel
problems or cancers would benefit from a good dose daily of
mother's milk!"

In Angelica Jacob's novel *Fermentation*, published in
London in 1997, the heroine has erotic dreams throughout
her pregnancy, which are stimulated by her growing desire
for strong cheese. She befriends a cheese merchant, an old
man in her village, who provides her, throughout her pregnancy, with different varieties to try. After giving birth she
decides to make some of her own.

Jacob writes:

The process was similar to massaging the teat of a
cow. I had to cup each breast in turn and tease the
milk out in drops until it flowed evenly. I placed the
milk in a bowl and when that was done the idea came
to me to make a small homemade cheese out of it.
The old man had given me some rennet and I stirred
this into my milk and then let the mixture set. After-
wards I tied the mixture up in a small muslin bag over
the sink and let it drip.

The cheese tasted mild and slightly watery. I
spread it on some bread and sprinkled salt over it to
bring out the flavour and when I had finished I lay
down on the bed with the child beside me in her cot.

After a series of chapters in which the protagonist's cheese-
tasting leads to disturbing dreams, this, the last cheese in

Jacob's story, is notable for its ability to produce peaceful-
ness and contentment—and a dream that eroticizes the
Annunciation.

The connection between breastmilk and good infant
health is clear-cut, but the ingestion of this mysterious fluid
also has undeniably spiritual ramifications within our adult
world—and not merely to us as parents. What scientists continue to measure, teasing out antibodies, fatty acids, and
interferon, poets continue to explore, delving into the "head
of dreams deeper than night and sleep," of "the calm milk-
giver," as Muriel Rukeyser writes.

In Christian mythology, breastfeeding and lactation are a
central metaphor for salvation and purity. One of the most
intriguing stories features the thirteenth-century "ascetic
mystic" Christina Mirabilis who, according to the scholar
Claire Phillips-Thoryn, fled to the forest after being tortured
and accused of being "possessed by demons." She survived
there alone for nine weeks purely on the breastmilk that spontaneously flowed from her virginal breasts. After being cap-
tured again, bound in heavy chains, and fed on bread and
water, her breasts again came to her aid. Phillips-Thoryn
quotes Mirabilis's biographer, Thomas De Cantimpre: "Her
virginal breasts began to flow with clear liquid of the clearest
oil and she took that liquid and used it as a flavouring for her
bread and ate it as food and smeared it on the wounds of her
festering limbs as ointment."

However precise our calculations, breastmilk, and the
women who produce it, will always be magic-seeming. As
Natalie Angier speculates, "If an adult were to drink human
milk every day, might that person grow huge, like Alice nib-

bling from the left side of the mushroom, or become immortal, like Hercules, say, or the vampire Nosferatu?"

The following story is told by an American man in his thirties, who was never breastfed as a child. He was keen to satisfy his curiosity, and offered to try making ice cream with breastmilk if I could help him acquire some. I approached a friend who was expecting a baby, and she agreed that if her breastfeeding went well, she'd be happy to donate some of her milk. A few months later they met over lunch and she handed him two packages of milk that she'd expressed for him: one containing breastmilk with medication in it, as she'd recently suffered a bout of mastitis, and one without. He then wrote to me about what happened, and the storm of feelings it occasioned. (His recipe is at the end of the book.)

Weave a circle round him thrice,
And close your eyes with holy dread,
For he on honey-dew hath fed,
And drunk the milk of Paradise.

—Samuel Taylor Coleridge, *Kubla Khan*

did it! After dinner, I was getting ready to throw it all out, and had decided, Well, I'm just going to have to let you down because this is too weird, and it's not fair that I should feel guilty for not doing something really weird. And then I had a change of heart wherein I simply felt, *Come on,* I want to know what this stuff tastes like, that's the thing, I want to know. And this was the genesis of the whole adventure, see, I just wanted to know what it tastes like. I tore open the end of the nonpenicillin package and just stuck my finger in there, and then I licked my finger. (I know, I'm giving you more details than you want.) It actually tasted *really good.* It's a little waterier than I thought it would be (well, it had separated a little bit too, since it had sat in the fridge for a whole day), but it's really sweet. I think my friend Danielle had it right: it tastes kind of like the milk left over in the cereal bowl. So there I was with this plastic bag full of this stuff, thinking of my friend Jennifer, that it had come out of her body somehow, and I had two very contradictory feelings, which is that it was intimate and erotic *and* really foul. I mean that I was both turned on and nauseated, literally nauseated, at the same time.

And yet I didn't want to waste the rest of what was in the bag, because Jennifer had gone to some trouble, and I just figured I could try to make some ice cream for the hell of it, and I could eat it, or someone could eat it, and that would be that. I was also sort of curious to see what kind of ice cream it would make. I wanted to know whether it had enough fat in it to make ice cream. I determined that I would forge ahead.

I found that Jennifer had given me three-quarters of a cup of mother's milk, which I bulked out with one quarter of a cup of organic skim milk. I added the requisite sugar and vanilla, and then, a little worried that it wouldn't gel properly, I threw in a raw egg (which is stupid, since this is how you get salmonella poisoning), beat the whole thing desultorily, and then poured it into the ice cream maker and went back to reading Flannery O'Connor stories for a while, not expecting much.

How surprising then that in ten or so minutes it was already hardening up! In the routine interval, which is about twenty minutes, there was, indeed, some ice-cream-like stuff going around and around in the rotating ice cream maker. So I busted it out of the machine and put it in a bowl, and then I ATE ICE CREAM MADE FROM JENNIFER'S BREASTS! There were about two servings of it, and it wasn't real ice cream, because of the absence of cream, but it was really sweet and tasted pretty much like that old ice milk that you used to be able to get (Light and Lively, it was called) in the seventies. Definitely icy but not creamy. I liked it. I ate about half, and then I started to feel like it might still be pretty fattening, especially if I ate it all, so I threw the rest out. And part of me was trying to get rid of the evidence.

Throughout, I felt that there was a strange ritual to all this, and that the ritual was sort of an attempt to comfort myself for the fact that I had never been breastfed myself. There was a symbology. There was some kind of consolation streaming down from the heavens, or perhaps just from my own imagination, for the fact that this intimacy had not been a part of my experience. Not that you can overcome such a thing in an evening. But the ritual of it seemed sorrowful, and interesting, and also taboo in some fundamental way.

I could never get clear of all the contradictory feelings. A little grossed out, but also intrigued. And I suppose I felt this amazing generosity of Jennifer to volunteer the substance, which is an understanding of motherhood that I never quite had before.

Cooking with Breastmilk

If you could cook with breastmilk, what would you make?

An omelet.

Cookies.

A banana-strawberry smoothie.

Mousse.

Breastmilk is for babies.

The most scrumptious, stinkiest, sharpest blue cheese—like
    Shropshire Blue.

Vanilla custard pudding.

Nothing! I hate cooking!

Vanilla ice cream with real vanilla beans.

A White Russian: vodka, Kahlua, and breastmilk.

Crème caramel.

I would add it to anything that has milk in it.

Face cream.

Mashed potatoes, laced with breastmilk, and served flat
    with multiple breast indentations.

Blancmange.

Urgh!

Café latté.

French toast, with cinnamon and brown sugar.

I wouldn't mix breastmilk into anything as it is already a
    complete food. All I'd do is water it down, as it is so
    intensely rich.

Indian style milky fudge.

Warm baked custard with freshly grated nutmeg on top.

I don't think I could cook anything with breastmilk. Out of the body is one thing, when it's fresh. But if it's been sitting in a glass, even for two minutes, I really don't want to have anything to do with it anymore.

In curries instead of coconut milk.

Hot chocolate.

White sauce for lasagna.

I'd serve it in a glass on its own, at room temperature. Anything else would disguise it.

Porridge.

Warm crème anglaise sauce, for a bread pudding.

Tres Leches cake—a traditional Mexican cake using three types of milk—evaporated, condensed, and whole. Add breastmilk to make *Quattro Leches* cake!

Eggnog.

Warm peach soufflé, with rasberry ice cream.

Rice pudding.

Pancakes, because they're sweet, and whenever we eat pancakes we are all having breakfast together as a family.

Mother's Milkshake, vanilla of course!

Breastmilk yogurt.

Marscapone.

Crème brulée.

Junket.

A Slippery Nipple: 2 oz. sambuca, 1 oz. Bailey's Irish Cream mixed with 1 oz. of breastmilk, 1 drop of grenadine. Pour sambuca into a glass. Layer in Bailey's mixture. Gently add a drop of grenadine to the center.

Thinking Through Breasts

⌒⌐〜

I n Isadora Duncan's autobiography, *My Life,* she tells of the early separation from her baby, who was only half-weaned. She writes, "Often when I danced, the milk overflowed, running down my tunic, and causing me much embarrassment. How difficult it is for a woman to have a career!"

Combining breastfeeding and a career is an issue close to the heart of many mothers. Where that career involves performance, as it did for Isadora Duncan, it is doubly challenging. Lactating breasts are not apt to dry up on cue. The image of a woman dancing, with milk running down her tunic, was for Isadora Duncan an embarrassing one. Yet it could also be seen as an image of great beauty, in which the harmony of flowing limbs and flowing milk could be expressed, in both senses of the term, simultaneously.

In her essay on breastmilk and dance, Barbara Browning writes, "Slowly we bend forward in a deep second-position plié, and Silvana guides our hands up our bodies, passing over our breasts and then flowing outward toward what was to be our audience. She reminds us that Yemanja created the oceans from her unending flow of breastmilk. As we repeat the gesture, I feel the incongruity of my hands running over my own diminutive breasts, trying to make this momentous, oceanic gesture. I have simultaneously the sense of my own smallness, and the magnitude of the movement in spite of that."

Performing a breastly dance onstage, trying to breastfeed a fractious baby in a restaurant, and making use throughout the working day of the few work-based pumping rooms are very different challenges. Most breastfeeding women have experienced some level of disapproval when feeding in public—from frowning glances to run-ins with shopping center management and even the police. As one woman recalled, in her reply to the questionnaire, about her shopping trip to Hong Kong with her three-month-old:

My concern was to do the right thing, so I rang Tourist Information on my arrival and they suggested that I would offend if I fed my baby in public, and should [therefore] do so in any toilets, or parent's rooms. Having this information didn't help, as I found out there are no parent's rooms, even in department stores. At the Ocean Terminal, which has a huge collection of shops for children, I asked one of the information people where I could feed my baby. She pointed to the chairs, and I then indicated "breast" by pointing to it, and her response was "Oh no, no, no, no! Come with me!" Well, she led me out the back of her office into a strange storage room with shelves and small wooden cubicles with various bits of luggage, she brought me a chair and faced it into the corner so I would be staring into this dark space, with no one walking through to see anything. She then brought me a whole roll of white toilet paper—to this day, I wonder what on earth for. Clearly I was not supposed to be seen by anyone.

Another woman who tandem-fed her twins discovered that even in a relatively tolerant environment, it just wasn't acceptable to feed, even in "a semipublic place at work." She writes, "It's all too flamboyant. There is absolutely no discreet way to tandem-feed twins, it's just tits-out, all the way." However, her experience has also been positive, as she writes later: "Breastfeeding has taught me to stick up for myself. You have two choices when you're sitting alone, feeding your baby, your breasts exposed for all the world to see, and a narrow-minded meathead with an agenda gets in your face. You can be ashamed, and hide yourself and your baby away, or you can sit tall and speak your mind, and let the world, and your baby, know that you are not ashamed."

The value of "sitting tall" has been demonstrated by women getting together to protest against harassment while breastfeeding in public. One of the best-known cases occurred in Connecticut in 1996, when a mother was ordered by a police officer to move on after stopping in a parking lot to breastfeed her baby. Incensed, she drove to the nearest police headquarters to complain, and later received an apology from the police department. Following this, she was joined by other mothers in the area as they staged a "breast-in" at a local deli.

As an organized response to this problem in Australia, it was decided that a competition would be held during World Breastfeeding Week, to challenge the *Guinness Book of Records* for the most women breastfeeding in the same place. In Sydney in 2001, a group of 536 breastfeeding mothers won a decisive victory over their runners-up in Western Australia, with 438 women. In 2002 this record was broken by a group of 1,130 women in Berkeley, California. Thanks to these sorts of events, legislation now exists in many states in both America and Australia to protect the freedom of mothers to breastfeed without harassment.

On Ariel Gore's website, *Hip Mama,* Gwen Zepeda wrote, "Here's how I see it: I'm going to feed my baby breastmilk when my baby is hungry, wherever I am. You might notice me doing so. Maybe, for some reason, it's not something you want to see. My suggestion to you is *turn your head the other way.* There. Now everyone's content. See how easy life can be?" Another woman told Ariel Gore, "I live to breastfeed, especially in public."

Men who are concerned about the protocol of the male gaze in the presence of a breastfeeding woman might adopt the advice given by Frank Moorhouse's character "the Former Mistress." Although admitting this is an area that can be fraught with complexity, after the narrator expresses his fear of being branded a perv, the Former Mistress cuts to the chase pleasantly by saying, "Go ahead, watch as much as you wish—don't keep averting your gaze with such deliberate casualness."

Although some men are clearly uncomfortable in the presence of breastfeeding mothers, I sometimes wonder if this is due to a misplaced sense of embarrassment on the woman's behalf. If men felt that women were more at ease, perhaps they would be too. We need to believe that just as mothers can separate their sexual lives from their maternal lives when necessary, so can fathers. This is echoed in one man's reply to the questionnaire, where he stated emphatically, "When I see women breastfeeding, I think of what a pure, innocent, and beautiful sight it is. I do *not* find it erotic. For me, it's a matter of nutrition and love, not sex—even though I'm a great and regular admirer of women's breasts."

Yet for others, the idea that a breastfeeding woman is sensually and emotionally satisfied can add to the pleasure of sharing her company while breastfeeding, particularly if she breastfeeds at the table and there is a sense of everyone sharing food together.

For Alison Bartlett, the writer of the following essay, work involves the performance of both her mind and her body, as a feminist academic and mother, and she shows how her lactating breasts have become central to the integration of her various selves. She raises several intriguing questions: How do lactating breasts fit onto the stage of the feminist thinker? How can the maternal body conduct its work within a patriarchy? And how can we perform our lives fully, as professionals and as mothers, making use of these experiences to become better at both?

As one woman wrote in reply to the questionnaire: "Breastfeeding is about relinquishing control, and that's a really scary and shocking thing to do when you are a strong and independent woman. For me, breastfeeding was about letting go, allowing chaos to come in and have a say about my life . . . it's shocking, and it's great."

At the same time, the intelligence of the breasts and the genius of breastfeeding have much to offer the workings of what we like to think of as the separate mind. Oliver Wendell Holmes perhaps put it too strongly when he stated, "The two hemispheres on the woman's chest wall will outwit the two hemispheres of the brain every time." As the midwives who use the term *milkbrain* to describe breastfeeding mothers well know, it's all mixed up together.

*B*ubbles of thought erupt through the subterranean swarm of seconds during my maternity leave. Words aren't remote, they're tumbling over each other, especially while I'm breastfeeding. Here I am, seated for hours, rocking, my daughter suckling and sleeping in my arms, my mind wandering between the profound and the trivial while engaged in this most profound and trivial of activities—this most corporeal of activities that insinuates itself into the most unimaginable places in my mind.

As a breastfeeding academic, I am bringing theoretical reflections to bear upon lived experience and embodied thought. I am complicating my relationship to ideas and memory, learning feelings, sensations, and practice.

In Kate Llewellyn's poem "Breasts," a woman's breasts are personified as readers and as knowers:

> *As I lean over to write*
> *one breast warm as a breast from the sun*
> *hangs over as if to read what I'm writing*
> *these breasts always want to know everything*
> *sometimes exploring the inside curve of my elbow*
> *sometimes measuring a man's hand*
> *lying still as a pond*
> *until he cannot feel he is holding anything*
> *but water*
> *then he dreams he is floating*

*

*in the morning my breast is refreshed
and wants to know something new*

But what can breasts know, and how do we know them? What can
breasts read, and how do we read them? These are matters that have
come to occupy my thoughts.

Breastly Dramas

I go to the theater with a newborn baby. The theater is at the university. It's opening night. The vice chancellor is there, along with other
important guests. I sit in a seat near the aisle so I can escape quickly if
my baby starts crying when she wakes. She wakes, and I offer her my
breast. She happily suckles for the rest of the play. I sit in the half-
light with my huge breast out, my daughter latched on. It feels curiously subversive. For what other reason could I sit in a theater with
one breast "exposed," unless performing maternity? It means mother
and baby don't disrupt the "real" performance, and yet some other
meaning is being disrupted, something to do with the way I've been
trained to behave in public.

Public Scenes

I am looking at the color photo taken by Annie Leibovitz of Jerry
Hall breastfeeding her son, Gabriel Jagger. It is a staged photo. The
model is wearing a little black dress with a tiger-striped fur coat over
it. She is fully made-up, wearing bright red lipstick, her long blonde
hair cascading over the fur. She is sitting cross-legged in a plush, red
upholstered chair, her body slightly side on, and we follow her long
legs down to see gold stilettos, and a gold chain attached with a heart
around her delicately curved ankle. The interior of the room is richly

furnished in red, black, and gold. It is a setting and a portrait position in which we might be used to seeing Jerry Hall placed, but the big naked baby in the very center of the photograph, suckling on a breast drawn out over the top of the dress, takes us by surprise. The baby is curled on her lap, one arm reaching up to the other breast; and he looks across his mother's body. Hall has one arm around her baby, protectively, supporting him, the other is draped along the chair as she strokes his foot. She looks directly at the camera, seriously, almost surly, daring us to challenge her.

In an American study of women's attitudes to breastfeeding in public, the sociologist Cindy Stearns refers to women "doing breastfeeding," and to "the possibilities for public performance." Due to cultural taboos and, in some states, legal sanctions, Stearns found that most women "proceeded with their breastfeeding as though it were deviant behavior," so that "being an invisible breastfeeding mother was the goal for many women."

Scandals

"Breasts are a scandal for patriarchy because they disrupt the border between motherhood and sexuality," writes the feminist philosopher Iris Marion Young.

I remember (another scene) nights sitting up in the dark breastfeeding through the pain of—bad positioning? unfamiliarity? soft nipples?—chanting to myself, Big strong nipple, big strong nipple, with tears quietly streaming down my cheek, and thinking, This is the pits. It can't get any worse.

As the pain becomes more intense through the night, I decide not to remain quiet but to vocalize the pain on each breath, making primitive animal-like groans while my daughter drowsily attaches and my partner sleeps on noisily beside me.

At some stage my babe discovers that I have two breasts, and while she suckles on one she stretches out her tiny hand to locate the other, softly caressing the curve of my breast, brushing past the nipple and then lingering over it, fondling the nipple and feeling it grow in her fingers. Like a lover but more tender, softer, smaller hands, but then rougher as she squeezes the nipple and I have to uncurl her fingers laughingly, squirming.

Listening to a women's radio program about breastfeeding I hear some women say they orgasm while breastfeeding their baby. Wow!

Breastspace

My breasts take up space. They stick out farther than before. They drift down more than ever, gently nudging my waist when I lean over, as if saddened somehow. They swing in a way they never used to. Friends tell me they will "settle down" after a while—as if they are excited.

I start to notice the way big-breasted women carry their breasts, what kinds of clothes they choose, their attitude in their posture, the amount of space they take up, and the ways their breasts move through the world.

Shopping Space

I discover a new space for my breasts: the parent's room. Recently added to many shopping centers and department stores, these rooms are competitively equipped with softly colored furnishings and decor, change tables, disposable towels. Some have toilets, others have microwaves, boiling water on tap, most have toys or a playpen. They're like a home away from home. They're so comfortable you can forget about the shopping center outside.

Almost. They're usually located right in the center of the center.

In fact, if the shopping center can be likened to an organism, the parent's room is located in its bowels, deep inside a labyrinth of pathways between entrance and exit. These secret inside passages conceal the activities of management, cleaners, defecation, and breastfeeding. Stearns's women would no doubt be grateful for such consideration, saved from the hostile public gaze. But I feel insulted, being locked away out of sight.

I sit in the café in the middle of the shopping mall to feed my babe.

Shopping for Breastspace

I go to Myer's department store to buy a maternity bra. This is what I'm supposed to do. It's part of the ritual of becoming a mother. I suspect it's also a way of strapping my breasts in, of confining them to the space they are supposed to occupy—out here, not down there. We three, the family trinity, stand and look at the rack of encased frames in sensible beige and washable nylon. They look ghastly. They are distinctly separated from the lacy, satiny, black, blue, red, *sexy* bras.

A Myer's lady comes to help. I try on three pairs and am horrified at the shape they make me, the coarseness of the fabric, the price, the utter nonsensuality of the thing. I feel pointy and stiff, the way Madonna parodies. I buy the least uncomfortable pairs on credit and flee. I rarely wear them. Sometimes if my breasts feel heavy and I want some assistance to hold them up, or if I go into work and feel as though I need protection, I put them on, like armor.

When I come home, I realize that I haven't been in touch with my breasts for many hours. The bras encase everything, including every feeling, so that I can't even tell when I'm full, when the ducts start to harden from engorgement. I get home and they're solid in parts. The bras disembody my breasts.

One day I dye the bras purple, but the various synthetic fabrics mean it is several shades of purple and they suddenly look old and worn. My bras died.

Breasts Unbound

I am reminded of the symbolism of bra-burning in the early public protests of 1960s women's liberation, which Iris Marion Young interprets as such: "Why is burning the bra the ultimate image of the radical subversion of the male-dominated order? Because unbound breasts show their fluid and changing shape; they do not remain the firm and stable objects that erotic fetishism desires. Unbound breasts make a mockery of the ideal of a 'perfect' breast."

And is it all the more scandalous, I wonder, for large, heavy, lactating breasts to be unbound? To go without nursing pads? To risk the possibility of leaking milk over clothes, leaving visible marks of maternity?

Outing

She's eight weeks old. A very different relation I have to my breasts now. I love to walk around with nothing on top. It's as if they need to stretch out and be aired in the open after being hoisted and protected and suckled and squashed. On Stradbroke Island I wander up the beach and take off my shirt, stretching out under the sun on my towel. It feels delicious.

I am taking my breasts to the beach. Sometimes it feels like they're on loan to me, they look so absurd on my body. I wonder how long they're here to stay.

The Language of Breasts

Coming to terms with breast changes was for me one of the central factors of making new meaning of myself as a mother. It's not necessary, though, to have experienced maternal breasts to be involved in negotiating breasts as a source of self-knowledge. As Iris Marion Young suggests in her essay "Breasted Experience," "few women in our society escape having to take some attitude toward the potentially objectifying regard of the other on her breasts." And, she adds, all women, whether mothers or not, "are still too often cast in the nurturant role." Many women who are diagnosed with breast cancer also feel impelled to examine the ways in which their subjectivity as women is connected with their breasts.

But it is the experience of my breasts as maternal that has intensified my relation to them. They became central to the ways in which I had to reinvent myself as a mother, in coming to terms with a new body and a new self, and have prompted my thinking through breasts.

Jane Gallop has argued that there is a significant difference between talking about "the breast," which functions symbolically, "like a painting in a museum," and "breasts," which are usually our own. In her essay "The Teacher's Breasts," she suggests that this difference is similar to the difference between phallus and penis. One is a cultural icon, the other a personal body part hidden from view. The ways in which we might talk about breasts, then, affect the meanings we're able to generate and use for ourselves.

Scene 1: Naming Breasts

One of my first dilemmas was what I wanted to call my breasts. There was always someone there to tell me that: "She wants some titty," "She's going for the boozie," "Where's the boobie?" "Time for breastie." The infantilizing gesture of adding a familiar *ie* to each term unnerved me for what were now these tirelessly active milk-filled parts of me.

Buxom is a word I feel inclined to employ in my feelings toward wearing these breasts, as well as *matronly*, a word both powerful and mute.

Scene 2: Keeping Abreast

Breasts loom curiously in figurative speech. *Making a clean breast of things* means "to make a full confession." But what is the meaning of a clean breast? And what is an unclean breast? Keeping something *close to the breast* often means "close to the heart," as is the left breast. I heard that babies often favor a woman's left breast because they're comforted by their closeness to the mother's heartbeat. Or is it because most people are right-handed? *Keeping abreast of things* is "to keep up, to keep in front." My dictionary also uses *breast* to mean "to face, meet boldly or advance against." These meanings are attached to the breasted position on the front of the body, as Kate Llewellyn's poem "Breasts" also shows:

> *as you will realise*
> *these are my body's curious fruit*
> *wanting to know everything*
> *always getting there first*
> *strange as white beetroot*
> *exotic as unicorns*
>
> *I know my breast knows more than I do*
> *prying hanging over fences*
> *observant as a neighbour*
> *or eager as a woman wanting to gossip*
> *they tell me nothing*
> *but they say quite a lot about me*

Scene 3: Breasts for Thought

Llewellyn's breasts are inquisitive. But there is a curious reference in my Penguin Macquarie Dictionary to "the bosom," which "is regarded as the seat of thoughts and feelings." Imagine that! "The seat of thoughts." Breasts as generators of ideas, as producers of knowledge.

Suddenly lactating breasts become fertile grounds of wisdom, active organs producing food for the mind as well as the body. What a difference this makes to the way breasts can be worn.

Writing Breasts

Breastmilk is just one aspect that constitutes the breast as a site of knowledge, or seat of thought. In her famously joyful essay, "The Laugh of the Medusa," Helene Cixous delights in the breast as a continually replenishing source of creativity that acknowledges "maternal debt"—the gift of maternity that can never be repaid and that our written culture struggles to acknowledge. Her controversial use of breastmilk as a means to write is uttered in the same breath as birth:

She gives birth. With the force of a lioness. Of a plant. Of a cosmogony. Of a woman. . . . And in the wake of the child, a squall of Breath! A longing for text! Confusion! What's come over her? A child! Paper! Intoxications! I'm brimming over! My breasts are too overflowing! Milk. Ink. Nursing time. And me? I'm hungry, too. The milky taste of ink!

I once tried taking her literally, but to write in breastmilk is to write in invisible ink.

Reading Breasts

I want to tell you about the textual relationship I have forged with my breasts. While I have been breastfeeding I have come to recognize that my breasts periodically act as barometers of my health and are driven to painful signals when "I" ignore my health. When I start to get rundown, my breasts register soreness at breastfeeds, and if I ignore those signals, they begin random stabs of pain during the day to bring my attention to them. "Help! Slow down! You're running yourself into the ground! Take notice or else!" they seem to say. Several times I've continued on with the anxiety of deadlines and lectures and had to take days off later to recover. If I respond promptly and rest, I recover quickly.

When I read back over the first year of mothering, it's always the times of stress and hurried life that coincide with breastly dramas. The last time it happened my daughter was eighteen months old. You'd have thought I would have learned to listen by then. Adrienne Rich's phrase, that "every woman is the presiding genius of her own body," makes a mockery of me.

The muscles of my breast then, as well as the fatty tissue, neurological impulses, vascular and endocrine system, are an embodiment of my physiological and psychological stress levels. I see capillaries of stress winding their way around my body, synapsing along with the message to increase milk production. My breasts are stressed. Me too.

My breasts and I are inseparable, coterminous. My breasts affect my thinking, my thought affects my breasts. Can we stretch our thinking to contemplate that breasts think?

To endow my breasts with "a field of knowledge" does not mean that I am always successful in making such knowledge legible, of reading or articulating such fields, as my breastly dramas illustrate. And such fields of body-knowledge are always subject to change, in the same way that my workload affected my experience of breast-feeding. But suggestions for an informed and knowledgeable body are tantalizing. My body has grown and birthed and nourished a child, its capacity to perform miracles of such magnitude is awesome, and rarely acknowledged in a medical system that claims authority and control over women's bodies. Even I forget this.

Imagine if breastfeeding was regarded as a form of bodily intelligence, if it was practiced with pride. Spines might straighten, shoulders might drop, necks might lengthen, and heads rise high, if breasts were worn boldly in all their shifting and unpredictable guises, visibly active, and even sometimes wet.

If we adopted Jerry Hall's defiant gaze to confront the camera's lens, what other shifts might this practice embody?

Moving Forward

For me, breastfeeding has not yet concluded, and so the questions continue. Like my breasts before me, I am pushing at limits, nudging at possibilities.

And so I take my breasts to work.

Pumping It

B reathless erotic celebration of the female breast is a well-known pastime in Western culture. We delight in being dwarfed by cleavages three stories high, beckoning like Sirens from inner-city billboards. We marvel at the bounce of well-endowed *Baywatch* stars as they prance along the beach in slow motion. Yet for all their generosity, the breasts that surround us, promising their gentle consolations to our neglected inner child, are sadly incomplete. They are Disneyfied, underwired, G-rated, and dry. Regardless of the amount of lace involved, they are bound and gagged—forever prevented from releasing their milk.

Full enough in one sense, though often technically nubile, the mainstream Western world's drought-stricken breasts are never skinny, but enticingly engorged and ripe. If they are surgically enhanced, their hardness and jut resemble the look of the breasts on a mother whose milk has just come in. They seem ready to explode, but they never do. Yet what if some of those Lycra animal prints pasted high up on buildings and scaffolds were to darken with moisture and drip slowly on pedestrians' heads? Would Franz Kafka have delighted in this surreal image? Would Philip Roth allow his mammoth fictional breast to shudder like blancmange as it heaved a sigh of relief? Would John Updike have his character Piet brush off his knees after climbing through the bathroom window in *Couples*, after reluctantly abandoning his lactating lover, and turn his face to the heavens, open-mouthed? Would we fear being flooded in one milky deluge, floating away like Alice in Wonderland on her own tears?

Perhaps a buxom classics scholar would raise her arms amid the joyous tumult and loudly recite from an ancient Egyptian love lyric: "Would you leave because you wish something to drink? Here, take my breasts! They are full to overflowing, and all for you!"

Perhaps the photographer David Lachapelle, whose *Milk Maidens* and *Naomi Campbell: Have You Seen Me?* are two rare exceptions to the rule of only celebrating the dry breast, would consent to creating such an image for a city billboard. Taking from the example of Antigua, Guatemala, perhaps we too could enliven our public spaces. Here in Parque Central is a fountain of a lactating woman, water for milk leaking through her fingers as she clasps her bare breasts.

Thankfully, there is a corner of our culture where the lactating breast is given its erotic, even athletic due. It is not socially acceptable. It is not well known. And it is a problematic and controversial field of work. But it can't be denied that certain soft-core erotica magazines and pornography videos do cater to a sizable market of people who desire leaky breasts. It turns out that there are gentlemen, and women, who prefer floppy breasts too, and fuller figures, and older partners. Some of these people need their fantasy of mothering to extend to a fantasy of nursing. Others revel in the joy of being sprayed by a woman's warm, sweet milk, or being forced to suckle.

In Susan Faludi's book *Stiffed*, published in 1999, she reports on the plight of male actors in pornography, who are paid significantly less than their female costars and often fail to achieve erections under the pressure of performing for the cameras (although the drug Viagra has since improved their lot). Faludi quotes Bill Margold, whom she describes as "a proponent of the in-the-toilet variety of porn," arguing why, ultimately, this lesser status of men in porn doesn't really count. He tells her, "The one thing a woman cannot do is ejaculate in the face of her partner. We have that power."

It wasn't until watching lactation pornography that I realized how untrue this is. Women can come in men's faces, too. And their milk lasts longer, sprays farther, and tastes better.

The following story is based on an interview with a pornography producer in the San Fernando Valley, Los Angeles. While I do not condone pornography that demeans or hurts its participants, whatever their sex, I am certain that images of women having fun with their lactating breasts—whether sexual, athletic, or slapstick—can help undo unnecessarily pious attitudes toward them, which keeps them hidden from view. For pornography featuring lactation begs the question: At what point in our history did the appearance of women's breastmilk become obscene?

It is Western puritanism that leads to disapproval of women nursing their children in public and contributes to the already long list of impediments to breastfeeding. It is not just because breastfeeding is seen as sexual that people object.

After all, we accept many public behaviors that touch on our sexuality, from eating and holding hands to kissing and the display of erotically charged body parts—slender ankles, smooth tanned thighs, heaving cleavages, and plumped up, reddened lips, to name a few. The concealment of breastfeeding also rests equally, if not more, on squeamishness relating to bodily function: the fact that food comes out of our bodies is an unsettling thought in a culture that rarely remembers that fruit grows on trees, or that cling-wrapped prime steak was once the rump of a cow. If we can imaginatively reconnect with the full physical potential of our bodies, and play with that knowledge, perhaps we can move away from alarm and panic toward honor and acceptance.

This is not to overlook the problems and pitfalls of working in pornography, or the evil of exploiting pregnant women in desperate financial straits. Unfortunately, it is only in pornography, and some rare examples of religious art, that alternative images of lactation are currently available. Nor is this to say we should enjoy all images of lactating breasts removed from the context of feeding babies. Some are funny, some are disturbing, some are Olympian, some are sublime. After a while, a lot of them are dull, which seems to me an okay development too. But many of the images celebrate and extend a real and complex aspect of female bodily expression.

I've been in this business since 1969. I was running a restaurant in L.A. that wasn't doing too well, and started developing motion picture films out the back. At one stage I'd thought I might become a chemist, so I had some background in chemistry, which was useful when it came to developing film.

I shot my first show in 1971, but my first lactation porn wasn't filmed until 1984, when I did *Battle of the Ultra Milkmaids.* It just kind of came along. There was this really cute girl, I forget her name now, who got pregnant and had these nice big hard breasts. I've always been interested in slightly offbeat ideas for shoots, so when I realized she was lactating I said, "Let's get that on camera."

The Battle of the Ultra Milkmaids sold really well, so then we did *Beyond the Battle of the Ultra Milkmaids.* Since then I've done the *Lactamania* series, which is now into eighteen volumes, as well as *Jersey Maids* and *Lactation Nation,* which is a compilation tape of best scenes. And we've done thirty volumes of *Ready to Drop,* which features the pregnant girls. I guess you could say we do about one lactation video a month out of sixteen tapes altogether, which is a small output compared to some companies, which might produce that many in one day.

My wife, Linda, runs the business side. We met in the early eighties when I was starting to distribute my own films. Linda had been working as a sales manager for an engineering company that sold parts to the government. I asked her one night over dinner how she felt about selling porno. She said, "What's porno?" But she figured if she could sell stuff to the government for millions of dollars then she could sell video.

The first company we formed was called Foreplay Video. Just the two of us sharing a single office with a closet for a stockroom. That didn't last too long. We now have several buildings and three distribution companies, Totally Tasteless, Hollywood Video, and Spunky Sperm.

We always did unusual material. We shot a lot of gay material that we distributed, which was a very good experience. We like anything that's a little bit off the beaten track. But I'd like to be remembered for shooting pregnant girls and lactating girls. That's the main thing.

I'd say I'm a maverick, and I'm thought of as risky. I do shows on the line. But I don't like to be extreme with women. There's no call for it. Although we do strange and unusual things once in a while, that's usually when a girl comes to me and says she wants to do it. In *Forced to Lactate,* there's some bondage element there, but the girls say it doesn't hurt.

I'm surprised by a lot of strange things—what people like. Not that lactation's strange. It's just one of those things you don't see every day.

Lactation porn is probably our fifth best-selling genre, coming after the *Aged to Perfection* series, which features women from forty to a hundred years. That's our number-one best-seller. Boobs would be two. Then it's a toss-up between lactation, legman's lassies, and cocks and frocks. There's a hat for every head.

Being on the set is fun. If you look at our cameras they're all covered with milk. I've used it in my coffee. In *Forced to Lactate,* we all put the women's milk in the coffee. In another title, we put milk in cereal and the girls ate it on film, as part of the story.

We nearly always use real milk in the films. Some of the girls have had breast implants, but they can still lactate. We do photographs every once in a while where we try different things. We did a photograph once of a girl with pierced nipples who wasn't lactating, so we put hypodermic needles through her piercings and shot milk out that way. But most of the stuff is real.

Most of the acting guys don't like the milk much. Some do. One of our star actors is a great lactation fan. He's a big bald guy, and you wouldn't want to meet him in a dark alley. But he's the biggest pussycat, and he loves the milk. The guys who do like it like the taste, they like the warmth. They like receiving from the woman, some of her bodily fluid.

But most of the guys are reminded of come, I think, or don't like the idea of being passive. You know, they'll say, "Oh, it's icky! Don't hit me with the milk!"

But I'm right in there. When I have to clean out all the glass tubing, sometimes it's a little strange. The milk goes a bit rancid. But otherwise it's fine.

When we're shooting, the atmosphere is fun. We make jokes. We make a mess. The milk ends up everywhere, all over the camera, all over the floor. We have a big piece of glass that we put over the lens so the girls can squirt directly into the camera. We get them to rub their nipples against it and smear the glass. We use a lot of mirrors too, and make a mess with them.

The only downside is when the girl dries up. There's only so much she can give at any given time. It's pot luck.

In *Jersey Maids,* we had the idea of getting the girls to sell their milk to rich men who could pay for it, even the president. The plot revolved around making deliveries to the White House. One of the Rockefellers used to drink women's milk in his old age. That's how we came up with the idea.

I think one of our best scenes is when I had this gigantic pump that I brought in from my garage. My editor, Eric Edwards, had this idea of lining up the girls and pumping, so I put together this tubing and equipment, which we attached to the girls. That was really spectacular. And the pump made this great *kathunka, kathunka, kathunk.* We had the girls sitting there polishing their nails, like in a beauty salon.

Then we've used my air power system, which I rigged up myself. The girls' milk goes into a big trough, and the milk trickles down into little tubes and into a bucket. Every drop is saved and we work it down. It's like liquid gold.

I also have a chemical pump that was probably used for pumping liquid from one place to another in a hospital operating room. Plus an antique Cleveden pump. I go to garage sales and secondhand stores, collecting things.

For example, I have what's called a thistle tube, which is connected to this shot glass with a rubber stopper. The thistle tube gets the milk going. I attach it to a Florence flask, which collects the milk from the thistle tube. The round part gives it a nice look.

I have lots of other ones too, really just wineglasses with the stems cut off. I've used a champagne flute too, which is good for a woman with small breasts, or someone who's kind of floppy. We've used standard breast pumps too, but I like these handmade ones.

We've used a manual pump, which is like a bicycle pump, or something for pumping up your backyard swimming pool. And a regular pump kit for a guy's penis. We did several scenes where the girl pumps the guy and then pumps herself. So they're both pumping.

If a girl comes to me and says she's lactating I get them to come and squirt for me before I bring them in for a shoot. So many girls say they can lactate, but they can't always produce much. Just a dribble. A lot of girls exaggerate, but then we're doing four scenes a day, which takes a lot of milk.

Some of them are supersoakers. Trinity de Loren was our first big one. She died of drugs a few years ago. She taught me how any girl can squirt milk by pushing on that little gland right behind your nipple. Every girl can do it. Some just a little bit. But you can do it.

I tell the girls to express milk for their babies the night before, so they're full of milk for the camera in the morning. I don't like having babies on the set because there may be legal problems. There's been a couple of times when the husband will bring the baby in halfway through the day for a feed, though, and then we start again.

I don't shoot for two weeks after the baby's born. Even though some of the girls want to. Some of them need the money. But I always make them take it off.

One of my girls went on lactating for a couple of years after she weaned, and continued shooting. It's popular because of the four scenes in a day they get to do, which is a couple of thousand dollars, compared to five hundred for one scene in a day, which is the usual deal. We do as much as possible because in a few months, a girl may not be lactating again, for the rest of her life.

The normal Adult video connoisseur gets jaded after a while. He always wants something different. But I think the main reason why men like the lactating girls has to do with mothering. It's what life and sex and the whole thing is all about. Pregnant women have always hidden their bodies, they've always been ashamed of themselves. But it's a beautiful thing. And most guys either nursed or wanted to. So it's ingrained in us, that need. It's not just older guys either. One of my lactating girls, Racquel, has started doing bachelor parties where she lactates as part of her act.

One of the great things about it is that we don't have to turn the girls upside down and do weird things with them. We don't pile-drive them, because we don't have to. If you have a cute little girl, people tend to do more and more disgusting dirty things with her to sell their video. Whereas if you have a pregnant girl or a lactating girl, you don't have to do that. The girl drives the show.

In the mainstream adult industry today, we've got a bunch of cookie-cutter girls that all look the same, all act the same, they're all pretty, cute, fantasy girl-next-door. That's not really where it's at, sexually. Where it's *really* at is pregnant girls, who *really* is the girl-next-door, or your wife, or any other attainable woman. We take the girl out of the fantasy and put her next door, or on the street with you. Especially pregnant girls with that glow. That's what sex is all about.

The Secret Life of Nipples

╲╭━━━╮╱

The *New Yorker* cover of November 27, 2000, features an illustration by Chris Ware, called *Thanksgiving.com*, which shows a futuristic New York City in which an outsize baby sits inside a high-rise building feeding herself via a tube attached to a feeding machine, not unlike the one that starred in Charlie Chaplin's film *Modern Times*. Through the window, the Chrysler tower and other well-known skyscrapers reach heavenward, while various flying machines drift past. Outside the room everything is pointy, tall, and thrusting. Inside, everything is round, molded to the body, and operated by switches or knobs. The feeding machine itself is nothing if not breastlike in proportion and shape.

The point the cartoon seems to be making (in addition to its high-tech alternative for avoiding the annual family drama of the Thanksgiving holiday) is that the technology that surrounds us is not entirely a product of masculine endeavor and wish fulfillment; nor does it always mimic the male body, as scholars like Camille Paglia might lead us to believe. Conversely, it suggests that the maternal function is not entirely natural either, but is also married to technology and culture.

This might seem self-evident to most women, whose bodies negotiate culture and technology every time they do up their bra, but it's amusing to see that images of female breasts in public spaces can still cause consternation in some quarters. In January 2002 U.S. Attorney General John Ashcroft spent $8,000 of taxpayers' money on drapes to cover the bared breast of *The Spirit of Justice*. This is an eighteen-foot aluminum statue of a woman gracing the Hall of Justice in Washington. It is clear that the marriage of women's curvaceous bodies and public life is still unaccepted in many quarters, despite the work of the Goddess Athena and Bodicea, not to mention Xena, Warrier Princess.

In response to the news of Ashcroft's cover-up, a poem was written by the American poet and playwright Claire Braz-Valentine. She writes:

> *John, John, John,*
> *you've got your priorities all wrong,*
> *While men fly airplanes into skyscrapers,*
> *dive bomb the Pentagon,*
> *. . . you are out buying yardage*
> *to save Americans*
> *from the appalling*
> *alarming, abominable*
> *aluminum alloy of evil,*
> *that terrible ten foot tin tittie.*

The spirit of Braz-Valentine's poem is echoed by the character in the following story, who speaks of the nipples' ongoing undercover work in eroding the worst excesses of patriarchy—or at least poking fun at them. The writer is a composite character based on replies to the questionnaire, research, and an old friend—a first-wave feminist, as open as she was voluble, who died several years ago in her nineties. In this story she is a grandmother and a psychotherapist who ponders what the nipple represents as a cultural icon. In the process, she comes up with some surprising uses for this prototype of all things technological, if not quite militaristic.

The prominence of the breast in early Greek religions would gradually be supplanted by what Eva Keuls has dubbed the "reign of the phallus."

—Marilyn Yalom, *A History of the Breast*

All babies have a passion for buttons. It is my duty to convince you of this fact. I'm a grandmother of four children, and raised two children of my own; and I've seen these children destroy—through sucking, biting, and twiddling —the entire row of many of my own pajama tops, plus many of their mother's and father's shirts, and, on one memorable occasion, my daughter's best friend's new designer jacket. True, buttons are close to a baby's mouth when it's being carried in an adult's arms, but so are fingers, jewelry, pens, chins, and collars. So let me tell you my theory about why this is so. I should also mention that I live in a somewhat unusual extended family, with my elder daughter and her two small children. Believe you me, I know their foibles.

Freud's definition of a *fetish*, put simply, is that it is the last thing a child sees before realizing its mother lacks a penis. I'm a retired psychotherapist, and my specialty was sexual dysfunction, so allow me to explain. In the process of a child's momentous discovery that its mother doesn't have a penis, the substitute object fixed upon by the child—that is, the fetish—takes on talismanic powers to ward off a fear of castration, in case the child too should end up as sadly unendowed as its mother. Put this way, it sounds a bit like the spell cast in *A Midsummer Night's Dream:* the first creature spied upon waking from the dream that his mother is genitally "complete" is the creature with which he is destined to fall in love. (The theory applies best to boys, and it was Freud's idea, which is why I'm using the pronoun *he* at this point.)

If this theory were literally true (and if the grandmother can stand in for the mother occasionally, which I can assure you, this one does), then my three-year-old granddaughter would almost certainly be in the thrall of a wooden spoon, as I remember precisely the moment she looked up at me while I showered, and how triumphantly she brandished this already much-loved kitchen utensil. Concerning her one-year-old sister, I am confident that she is yet to part with her belief that I am perfectly all and everything, just like all her adult carers, an entirely self-sufficient universe outside of which nothing of importance exists.

Not wanting to belittle Freud's efforts, it seems to me that a child's button fetish is based not on the last thing she sees before coming to terms with her mother's tragic loss. To my mind, it is the very *first thing* she sees, and feels and fondles, and masters, and makes use of. A mother's nipples are the things any child knows best on her mother's body, and perhaps, at a certain stage of children's development, the things they know best in the world, full stop. Having sucked and played with them for hours and hours, and for several years in some cases, they see them as cute and funny playthings, like a well-used favorite toy, the source of all diversion, pleasure, comfort, and, let's not forget, milk. Of course, if a child isn't breastfed, then the mother's nipple will be replicated by the latex or rubber teat on the child's bottle, and will still be an object of supreme importance in the child's young life.

It seems to me, on looking into the nature of this button obsession—which is a child's first habit, if you discount the suckling activity itself—that there are nipple substitutes for all of us, everywhere. From our first exposure as infants—either literally, to our mother's nipples if we were breastfed, or figuratively, to teats if we were not—many of us have covertly carried this passion for buttons into adulthood. There are even cases of button phobias, with one of my patients reporting fainting spells when she chanced upon small round pearl buttons in particular. This is the exception that proves my point: For most of us, nipples are impossible to resist. And whether we make use of the myriad substitutes surrounding us, or hold out for the genuine article, their compulsive appeal is undeniable.

Like it or not, button interaction is *everyone's* modern-day habit, not just children's. If you care to pause and look in detail at the surface of your daily life, you will see that it is densely populated with nipple symbols and substitutes, like mollusks on a seaside rock. Phallic symbols abound too, of course, with tall buildings, space missiles, joy sticks, and asparagus spears all continuing to enjoy their day in the sun. But nipple symbols are far more plentiful, and in tactile terms, they are much closer to our everyday lives. It is as if the humanoid's opposable thumbs were invented just for this. From fastening our shirts in the morning to turning out the bedside light, there is little we do without making use of these knobs and switches.

Moreover, it is the button that now makes this skill so necessary to survival. The further advanced we are technologically, the more plentiful these nipple substitutes have become. And who put the *tit* in *substitute* to start with, might I inquire? Oh, I love a pun, don't you? My late husband used to ask me, whenever he wanted sex, "Are you feeling cuntable?" I couldn't resist him!

Let me see, where was I? Oh, and it's not just at work that these buttons abound, exercising our opposable thumbs all day long. Art too relies on this pincer grip action, as it's called. Almost all musical instruments work on a similar principle of button or key pressing, while wind instruments add the oral dimension of sucking and blowing—a pure, albeit disciplined, mammary indulgence requiring years of practice.

Consider the commonness of the computer keyboard, with all its little finger-sized keys to press, and designed specifically so all fingers can optimize their contact, although I know many of you limit yourselves to your two index fingers, which is a shame. Then there's the computer keyboard's extension, the curvaceous mouse, with two smooth buttons at its summit—a full breast and two nipples in one elegant whole, ergonomically molded to the human hand. Think of the comfort this affords office workers during moments of stress, when they can grasp this soothing object.

And for those who use portable computers, how sensual the tracings of one's index finger across the responsive membrane of the track pad! Like a breast, it responds best to a delicate but sure touch. Poking, tentativeness, or brute strength will get you nowhere, just as I so often used to advise my patients.

And while we're on this subject, let's heartily condemn Toshiba's tracking button. Nestled in the keys, between *G* and *H,* it fails because it resembles a clitoris rather than a nipple. It's an annoying green nub—wobbly, and contrarian, and prone to causing hand cramps. Like masturbating on Prozac.

If this silly knob is an example of a button gone wrong, it is just another exception to remind us that buttons, in general, have been honed to perfection. Designers of high-tech gadgets now agree that buttons can't be smaller than the average human fingertip, or they cease to be useful. A useful button can possibly be no smaller than the hood of a clitoris, to tell the truth (which is why the Toshiba knob fails, since it is smaller even than that). And definitely no smaller than one's average nonengorged nipple. Take the common home-based remote control, for example, which has become button central of our domestic lives, its popularity casting the humble dildo into obscurity. Also the calculator, and banking machines. Light switches and tele-phone dial pads. Even toilet flushers, which, when I was young, were wooden handles dangling on the end of a long chain, but are now dis-crete round silver buttons requiring the merest pressure of the finger-tip. Then there are cigarette lighters that pop out of dashboards, or Bic and Zippo pocket lighters. And take a sheet of bubble wrap in your two hands. It is impossible to resist popping it, one bubble at a time, until the entire sheet has been cruelly deflated.

Doorbells also ask to be pressed, as knockers demand to be fondled. (Pun intended, of course!) Then there's the vending machine, its pro-grammable pregnancies giving endless birth to potato chips, soft drinks, and cigarettes. Plus the control panels of almost everything, from dishwashers to nuclear reactors. Hot buttons, panic buttons. And, during the cold war, simply The Button, which, like any self-respecting matriarch, could instigate World War III and destroy the planet.

The human nipple is the *über* switch. It is a physical prototype of all our technology for connection and for using a small effort in one place to produce a large result in another. The nipple demonstrates how stimulation in one field of activity results in a reaction elsewhere. Press it, pull it, suck it, or fondle it, and an objective is achieved in another region of endeavor. When a baby suckles, the pituitary gland releases prolactin, the milk-producing hormone, and oxytocin, which triggers letdown, and the milk begins to flow. When a lover fondles, oxytocin floods the body, resulting in sexual arousal of the genitals, a phenomenon reported by both males and females. One of the most interesting cases I ever had was a male patient who had an astonishing facility to reach orgasm simply by having his nipples fondled. Sadly, he could get few of his women partners to do this for him, since they saw it as a feminine desire, as if their own tricks were being plagiarized. The therapist he saw before me—a man, of course—was even less helpful than his girlfriends, and told him, "Men don't have breasts! They have chests!" All I could do was reassure this patient of his own good luck.

Let me see, where was I? Oh yes, we live in an age of small things becoming smaller, as though all these buttons—made of plastic or steel or whatever new materials are emerging—have erectile tissue that tightens and concentrates its powers of response the more it is tweaked. In view of this, I was not surprised to discover that in 1795, at the dawn of the industrial revolution, women in Paris wore their breasts proudly exposed beneath the transparent bodices of high-waisted gowns. A historian could be forgiven for interpreting this as a prematurely nostalgic longing for all things pastoral. But it's clear that these women were demonstrating a shift in uses of the body—not just its imminent redundancy in the face of automation, which promised to free it for pleasure, but its use as a design template for those very machines that would put it out of work. And take the common champagne glass, invented a few years earlier when Louis XIV placated a jealous mistress by using one of her breasts as a mold to cast a new vessel from which to sip his finest Krug. From this point on, the breast has been the true symbol of modernity.

Needless to say, there is a rampant orality contained in this sparkling image of a champagne glass (impractical though it turned out to be compared to the flute, its more vaginal counterpart). And so there are countless examples of oral gratification that act out our longing for reunion with the maternal breast: pulling on cigarettes, sucking on cigars; sipping from small apertures in round cans, or sucking more vigorously through a straw. It seems no small coincidence that the words *nibbles* and *nipples* are so phonetically close— also a *nip*, the smallest possible measure of strong liquor. Think of the irresistible hand-to-mouth nibbling and finger-licking required for the full appreciation of pretzels or popcorn. And think how many bored students have nibbled ruminatively on the nipple of a ballpoint pen, or—even more satisfying—*click, click, clicked* on the button of their retractable PaperMate with fingers or teeth.

Since we're on to pens, let's look briefly at their future. Once regarded as the genteel phallic symbol, they do seem to be on their way out, at least in relative terms. The pen is no longer mightier than the sword, if it ever was, since it was certainly never as mighty as the button. Even in the days of handwritten messages that might result in the death of the messenger, it was the wax seal, a small round signature, that proved the legitimacy of the document. Everyone knows that warfare is now performed at the press of a button. And even if a projectile might be involved from time to time, it's the finger on the trigger that sets it off. The quill is barely a memory, and the faint association between semen and ink must scarcely register any longer in the technological unconscious.

Looking at today's technology for cursive handwriting, the most useful development recently has been in the addition of cushiony finger grips, reminding me of the one maternal feature of the erect penis—its spongy, might I suggest bosomy, head. References to arrows and spears are done for. Softness and comfort are the order of the day. And so I pose the question: Is this the phallic gone explicit, hoping to pull up its britches by replicating itself in our handheld world in anatomically correct outline? Or could it be possible to imagine that there might be some androgynous integration of the two sexes' genitals on the way?

And so to conclude, while the phallic sailing ship undeniably thrust its hull through the high seas into new worlds, and the rocket ship thrust its nose into far-off galaxies, it was, and still is, the controls onboard these vessels, becoming smaller and smaller through time, that guided their path. And might I add, the ongoing obsession of young women to acquire an enormous bosom, using cosmetic surgery and uplift bras, can only mean one thing: The breast has become the new phallus. The breast is the caring erection, proving once and for all that women make the most important contributions to our culture. And were we to acknowledge the female phallus's power to give forth a stream of lifegiving fluid from within, its old adversary, the male phallus, would have to seriously consider an amicable detente, or risk being crushed forever.

The Place of Breastfeeding

If breastfeeding were a place, what would it look like?

A bed.

The Bahamas.

A pillow.

A beanbag.

Anywhere on CNN, at three in the morning.

A big red rocking chair.

The cocoon of a silk moth.

A Japanese garden.

A sparkling lake.

The Pantheon, whitewashed and heated.

Cotton-wool clouds.

A temple.

A forest.

A cave.

Warm waters.

Heaven.

A duvet.

My blue sofa on a rainy day.

A dairy.

A desert island.

My bedroom in the morning.

A sunny field in spring.

A hospital room with a nurse standing over my shoulder
saying, "A little to the right. Straighten that shoulder.
Keep the mouth open and the tongue down."

A park bench near a winding river.

A hammock.

The bath.

A log cabin, with a fire going and a table laden with food
and drink in the middle of a blizzard.

The place of humanity.

A circus.

The summit of a mountain—and all I can see all around
and beyond is wilder than anything I ever imagined.

That Sense of Yes

〜◦〜

While researching this book I came across several claims of men breastfeeding their own children, but I've never had the pleasure of witnessing this event. In her essay "Milkmen: Fathers Who Breastfeed," Laura Shanley tells how she conducted an experiment with her husband, David, when they had their first child, to see if he could lactate. She writes, "He began telling himself that he could lactate, and within a week, one of his breasts swelled up and milk began dripping out."

Although David decided not to breastfeed their baby, Shanley went on to research the subject and came across a number of cases of breastfeeding fathers documented by anthropologists and historians. Her examples include a fifty-five-year-old Baltimore man, mentioned by the nineteenth-century German explorer Alexander Freiherr von Humboldt, who wet-nursed the children of his mistress; and a South American peasant whose wife fell sick after delivery, so he breastfed his baby exclusively for five months.

The Christian Apocrypha also includes lactating men, as in Clare's dream of Saint Francis, in which he bares his breast and says to her, "Come, take and drink." Christ too uses breastfeeding as a metaphor for spiritual sustenance when he says, "Whosoever thirsteth, let him come to me and drink." Although these are no doubt metaphorical instances of male lactation, they suggest that men throughout history have at least imagined their breasts as nurturing.

In her essay Shanley quotes an anecdote from a friend about a gay couple in America who adopted a friend's baby and breastfed her exclusively for eight months. Shanley's friend writes, "By the time the baby was twelve weeks old he was making a full milk supply! He stayed home with the baby (he was a massage therapist). . . . I don't think many people outside their intimate circle knew about it, I'm sure folks would have had a fit if they'd known. . . ."

After reading her essay, I contacted Laura, and she subsequently put me in touch with an Englishman, now in his late fifties, who said he'd lactated sufficiently to help his wife breastfeed their second child in the 1970s. He wrote, "We wondered if it were possible for a man to breastfeed. I am a little on the chunky side and had small breasts. We were successful to a degree although I did have to supplement my feedings with expressed milk."

Laura also sent me an email from another man, written a year before, in response to her article. It read: "Laura, I was glad to see your article on milkmen. I was able to help my wife breastfeed our twins back in 1996. Getting my milk established took a long time and a lot of believing that I could actually do it; but after eighteen weeks I was able to feed one baby three times a day."

In Jared Diamond's 1995 article "Father's Milk," published in *Discover,* he writes, "We've known for some time that many male mammals, including some men, can undergo breast development and lactate under special conditions. . . . Lactation, then, lies within a male mammal's physiological reach." He notes that lactation in men (and women) can be a side effect of certain tranquilizers or other medications that affect the pituitary gland, as well as certain kinds of surgery that stimulate "the nerves related to the suckling reflex." He also notes that "Mere repeated mechanical stimulation of the nipples suffices in some cases."

In *The Emperor's Embrace: Reflections on Animal Families and Fatherhood,* Jeffrey Masson also provides a comprehensive picture of the many ways in which male animals—from beavers and penguins to turkeys and wolves—contribute to parenting, in some cases using their bodies to provide "milk" for their young. He suggests that the human male might learn from some of these examples.

While it's possible that a man might go to the trouble to help his partner breastfeed their children, it's hard to imagine that many would be highly motivated to do so. Harder still to imagine a sample large enough for a study of the components of male breastmilk compared with female breastmilk. It's known, for example, that women who induce lactation for their adopted babies do not produce colostrum. What other variations might exist, for better or worse, between women's and men's milk?

From the evolutionary point of view, there's been little reason for men to breastfeed, since human offspring can survive with the care of one parent, and it was impossible until recently, with the advent of DNA testing, to guarantee that a child was fathered by any given male. But with DNA testing and the use of fertility drugs leading to multiple births, Diamond imagines that a time might come when this will change. "Soon," he writes, "some combination of manual nipple stimulation and hormone injections may develop the confident expectant father's latent potential to make milk. . . . It wouldn't surprise me if some of my younger male colleagues, and surely men of my son's generation, exploit their opportunity to nurse their children."

Diamond wonders if there will still be a psychological hurdle to jump, considering that breastfeeding is viewed as a woman's job. But this might not just come from men shy of expressing their feminine side; it could also come from women fearful of men muscling in on their territory. When I showed the following story to one of my friends, she was concerned that men might take over, turning the whole culture of breastfeeding into a competitive sport or, more insidiously, undermining women's superior contribution to child rearing. Such reasoning fails to acknowledge how hard it would be to keep men ignorant of the downside, such as pain, cracked nipples, and engorgement.

On the other hand, if men suffered these problems, perhaps they would be taken more seriously. As Gloria Steinem speculated when she wrote "If Men Could Menstruate," research into the medical treatment of any problems men experienced would suddenly be hugely well funded. Not to mention that there'd be competitions in supply records. Shanley's website includes an illustration of a lactating man in *Emblematic Figures* by sculptor Giulio Romano (1492–1546). It shows him producing not just a spray or a trickle of milk, but a gushing stream, from his left breast. Just as Steinem predicted, "Men would brag about how long and how much."

More realistically, though, and in contrast to the fear of competition, there is the opportunity of spreading the load. The man who tells the following story did not, to his knowledge, produce milk. Nor did this bother him. But in offering his breast to his baby daughter, he is certain his experience helped him to become a more caring and effective parent—a prospect that no overburdened mother could readily disapprove of. As Shanley says, "I suddenly remembered my mother telling me years ago that as an infant I once tried to nurse on my father. I laughed about it at the time, yet I'm sure it is a fairly common occurrence. Babies want to be loved, nursed and nurtured. The gender of the person doing it is not important."

German academic Barbara Sichtermann, writing on "The Lost Eroticism of the Breasts," also points out how this sharing of the load can benefit fathers: "This is where I see men playing a part in caring for babies at any rate. We women can and must put pressure on men, force them to take on some of the duties involved in looking after children. It is essential that these duties are shared if women are to win equality in any other field. But we can also *win over* the men by offering them a share in pleasure. Babies are looking for food and comfort from the breast—and they could get comfort just as well from the fine and sensitive breasts of men."

Just as breasts create a bridge between mother and child, perhaps, since both sexes have them, they could also create a bridge between men and women.

She had Scully's heart whamming in her ear like a bell, like God singing.

—Tim Winton, *The Riders*

This is a story about Miyuki, who is my third child, and my second daughter. When my first two children were born I was studying, so I didn't spend much time at home during the day. But with my second marriage, Naomi started working shortly after she had our first baby, and I stayed at home. I was building extensions on the house, so it was quite easy to look after Miyuki. Every day I'd drop Naomi off where she worked at an opal store in the city, and then I'd feed the baby Naomi's expressed milk during the day before going in to collect her in the late afternoon.

But one day Naomi had driven into work. She was supposed to finish early, but she was late, and we'd finished all the expressed milk. It was unbearably hot, and I was walking round the house wearing only a sarong. Miyuki was frantic, so I was cuddling her, and patting her, and trying to get her to stop crying. She was very strong. When she cried the whole street knew. And she wouldn't stop until she got what she wanted. I was almost beside myself. She was throwing her head from side to side, then at one point she brushed against my nipple, and latched on.

I was a bit shocked by this but not as much as Miyuki was. Her eyes opened really wide and she looked up at me in surprise. Then she took herself off my breast, and her tongue was coming up and off her lips, and she was a bit confused, because I've got a few hairs around my nipple and naturally enough Naomi doesn't have any. I've only got about five hairs—a bit like Homer Simpson's head—but this was five more than Miyuki was expecting. She obviously thought, Something's dreadfully wrong here, dreadfully wrong. But she'd stopped crying.

So I thought, Okay, maybe this is a good idea. And I just gently lifted her head back up against my nipple, and she attached again, and looked up at me, and started sucking.

That look of confusion on her face is such a lovely memory. That little jar in her mind that something's not quite right. You can see she's thinking, Everything's going along fine, but something's changed. There was real consternation too. Then the idea started to crystallize that Yes, you'll do. So she'd suck a bit, then stop, and then she'd take her head off and look up at me, and look at my nipple, and look back up at me, and then go again, but a bit more tentatively. I think she was still trying to work out what the hell was going on.

At first it was a little painful. But it was a strange feeling. It was a mixture of Well, this is better than her crying, but should I be doing this? What if the neighbors see? But the relief of having her settled in such a short time, compared to what we'd been through for the past hour, just overcame everything. Even if some people might think it was wrong, it quickly became clear to me that this was what I should be doing.

It made me realize how arbitrary some of our customs are. I can walk down the street without a shirt on, no problem. I would never have discovered I could nurse Miyuki if I hadn't been wearing only a sarong that day. And Naomi, because of changes in our culture, is now able to breastfeed a baby in public as long as she does it dis-

192 • Fresh Milk

creetly. But if I were to breastfeed Miyuki in public, it would cause an uproar. And yet here is a nipple that's sanctioned for public viewing. I'm just not allowed to do anything with it.

The pain didn't last. The first time it was more of a surprise really, because it's an area of my body that's usually neglected. The only other time my nipples ever bothered me was when I was a surfer. You get the sand in the board wax and you're constantly rubbing up against it, so my nipples would get very sore and I'd end up with dreadful board rash.

It also reminded me of a drug I was taking when I had bad acne. I was about sixteen, and the skin specialist I was seeing put me on these pills. I'd been taking them for a while when I noticed that one of my nipples was getting hard. So the next time I went back to see him, which was once every few months, he said, "How are the pills going?" I said, "They're going really well, but one of my nipples has gotten very hard."

He went pale and fumbled a bit and said, "Well, I think we'll change those pills now because I don't think as a sixteen-year-old you really want to start developing breasts." He had put me on steroids.

When I was looking after Miyuki I started to wonder if I took those pills again there'd be a better value for her or what? It really crossed my mind that maybe I could take it a bit further. I mean, men's nipples always seem so superfluous, don't they? Maybe they could be more useful.

So it became a common thing. If Naomi was going to be late, I knew that there was always something there. If I'd run out of Naomi's milk, and Miyuki wouldn't suck on a piece of apple in a stocking or play with an ice cube, there was always my breast.

It became my sort of last ditch, and then my sort of not-so-last ditch, until it became just another reasonable way to not let her get too upset. She'd still be a bit confused at first, but then she'd look up at me and carry on. It obviously soothed her. So I just let it go.

I always used my left breast. Probably because I'm right-handed. And I guess the sound of my heartbeat might have helped to calm her down. It was one of those things that just happened.

She was still breastfeeding when she was two years old. But I wasn't! One or two bites with the teeth cured me of that. We stopped before her first birthday. And Naomi had stopped working by then, so it wasn't an issue.

One afternoon before then I was sitting in our Volkswagen van, waiting for Naomi, who was busy at her shop. Miyuki had been going off for about fifteen minutes, so I just took her out of her baby capsule and sat her on my lap. Sitting up in the front seat of a Volkswagen van, you get a very good view of the driver from the outside, but I was more concerned with getting her settled than how things might look. So I pulled up my T-shirt and held her, and she attached herself as usual and started sucking. By this stage we'd done it a number of times. She wasn't confused, and she'd simply latch on and suck, and look up at me and relax. We were old pros. It was so nice. That look she would give me at these times was incredible.

Just as we were settling down, a busload of Japanese tourists were leaving Naomi's opal shop and walking past my van to where their tour bus was parked just up the road. We'd been there for about five minutes when suddenly I realized that right in front of us, just a few feet away, a group of people had stopped. The first five had started walking past the van and glanced over and stopped cold in their tracks. Their eyes were wide open. Then there was a concertina effect as everybody else behind banged into them until there was this little huddle of people, about thirty or so, staring in disbelief at this man sitting in his van, breastfeeding a baby. They were open-mouthed. They couldn't take another step. No one spoke. No one pointed. They were transfixed.

I think the greatest shock came when Naomi, who is also Japanese, came out of the shop, raced across the road, passed her customers of ten minutes earlier, jumped into the van, and grabbed the baby. In one motion the baby came over, the top came up, the bra came down, the baby was now attached to her. The people just stumbled off.

When the bus drove by a few minutes later, all their faces pointed out the window, silently checking that it could possibly have been true.

I think if men lactated it would improve relationships between fathers and their children. I considered myself at that time a very experienced parent, having two older children who were then nine and seven. But this was different. This was a real confidence that I was enough, at least until Naomi could be there.

Breastfeeding would also make many men more comfortable handling babies. One thing I noticed with men, and probably with me at first, is that men's interaction with babies is like their behavior with toys. They'll play with the baby and they'll stimulate the baby and expect it to respond in a lively way. It all happens at arm's length. Those quiet moments of intimacy are not there. If men could lactate and share the feeding, and share in those early stages of development by providing not just the physical well-being as far as food and nutrients are concerned, but also that sense of safety and security, I think it would change a lot of things.

When Miyuki first latched on, I understood that this child was a part of me. Instead of just being the father of the child, she was a part of me. It made me feel a little bit more complete. It's something that's stayed with me.

It's only when you hold a baby at your breast that your gaze can lock. You can't do this and not lock eyes and scan each other's faces. Your whole world becomes that little circle of the face, and sounds drift off. And in that stillness and safety you can really see. Once she was attached, and looking up at me, I found it very difficult to look away because of that connection, that sense of yes.

As we got better at it, it was less intense. She'd suck for ages, and some afternoons I could just sit down and watch a whole TV show, and she'd occupy herself at my breast. By that stage we could just while away our time together.

When I relate the story of that closeness between Miyuki and me, I'm always reminded of that look she'd give me when she latched on, and the feeling of her whole body relaxing against mine. From being a tense and dissatisfied baby, she would melt into this soft bundle. It was safe. We were close.

Of course, as soon as Naomi was there, I had no hope of breastfeeding, because Miyuki would know right away. She could probably smell her. She would be like, "I don't want second best—I know the other stuff's here somewhere."

But Naomi thought it was a good idea. And we both thought it was funny. I used to say to her, "I'm a bit sore today. Why were you so late?"

We were relieved too, because it had been an awful period of time, that half an hour in the afternoon, which I'd dreaded, hoping Naomi wouldn't be late. Before we discovered this, I felt there was absolutely nothing I could do. I couldn't take her for a walk. I couldn't solve the problem. It seemed unfair that I didn't have that mechanism to provide for her. I'd always watched the other two being fed and used to think, Gee, you're so lucky because even if the child is not hungry but is upset, it will be quite happy to suck and be satisfied.

Of course, I've also seen the downside. I've seen the cold cabbage leaves. I've seen the swelling and sensed the burning. But it's such an easy, soothing device, and one that the giver can also receive a great deal from. It can soothe you, the carer, whoever you are.

I guess there's no way to quantify how it's shaped our relationship. But I'm sure it must have. Perhaps she's a little more trusting of me, by going through all the things we've been going through, moving across the country to Melbourne from Perth, and knowing that everything will be okay. She seemed to accept it rather well. She accepts me.

Since Miyuki was a baby, one thing we've done together is watch planes. It started in Perth, when I'd drop Naomi off at work in the morning, then Miyuki and I would go and have a coffee, and on the way home we'd drive by Perth Airport, around the perimeter fence, and walk down to watch the planes. We'd stand about a hundred meters from the end of the runway and the planes would take off and land over us. When she was little, I'd cradle her in my arms and cover her ears.

It's amazing. When the 747s are full, they use up all the runway. They'd be about fifty or sixty meters up. It's a real test of your faith in aeronautical engineering. When they're landing you can hear the sound of the air whistling through the engines. Miyuki thought it was fantastic.

When she was older, and I took both her and Kim, her younger brother, and he was frightened, I'd say, "It's okay, Kim, you're safe."

And Miyuki would say, "Yes, if Daddy says it's safe, it's safe."

Miyuki is seven now, and often when she sits on my lap while we're watching TV I can remember that closeness, even though it's not there anymore in that intense way. And I'll just look at her, and she'll say, "What? What?" And I'll say, "Oh, nothing. I'm just remembering something from when you were a baby."

I will tell her one day, perhaps when it's her turn to feed a hungry child.

Feeding Triplets

I received only a couple of replies to the questionnaire that referred in passing to the daunting task of feeding twins. Perhaps mothers with multiples are too busy to answer questionnaires. Then I spoke with one woman whose memory of the pain and exhaustion from feeding twins was still vivid five years later. My offer of a free drink was not enough to induce her to think about it again.

One midwife told me of her awe and amazement watching how a mother of triplets managed to breastfeed. At each session she would feed the first child from one breast, the second child from the other breast, and then the third child from both breasts. With the organization of a military campaign she would keep track of this schedule and rotate it.

Another midwife told me the little-known fact that all mothers who breastfeed initially produce enough milk for two children—even if they give birth to only one child. Women are often exasperated with the process of breastfeeding when they become engorged in the first few weeks, as though the body were dimwitted. But in reality the body is being smart, as it initially makes enough for twins, or perhaps for older siblings, in case it's needed, before settling into the right amount. One woman who breastfed her twins spoke of the importance of trusting that she could produce enough milk, and developing what she called her "milky mentality." This worked so well that she soon had plenty for her twins and "enough left over for the whole street."

The intelligence of the body is demonstrated by mothers who tandem-feed—that is, they breastfeed a newborn together with an older sibling who is yet to be weaned. They are advised before giving birth to keep the toddler on one side and allow the other breast to dry up slightly so that it produces more colostrum. (As any child is weaned, the breasts produce colostrum again, so that the child receives an extra dose of antibodies before moving on.) If the second breast has been allowed to regress this way, the mother's milk supply will increase more rapidly after she gives birth—in twenty-four hours, rather than the usual sixty hours. Once the baby has established feeding, the mother can then proceed to feed both her children from both breasts.

One mother's experience of breastfeeding twins was so empowering and positive she subsequently changed careers and became a lactation consultant. She recounted the following story: "My strongest memory is the amazing pleasure of looking down at both my babies feeding and playing fingers with each other during a feed. No one else saw them from this perspective. This vision simply belongs to me and me alone."

She too commented on the importance of positive thinking when faced with the challenge of feeding more than one baby. "Two instances are fixed in my mind," she recalled. "One was the negative effect of a midwife commenting when

I took my expressed milk into the nursery, 'Is that all you have?' The second was the clinic sister who always said, 'That little girl is starving her brother,' as my daughter put on stacks of weight and my son plenty, but not in comparison to her. I found professional support [twenty-five years ago] about my decision to breastfeed lacking."

She also pointed out the advantage of having twins when they choose to wean themselves abruptly. "I clearly remember my son at twelve months, biting me, sliding off the lounge, and never asking for another feed. His twin sister continued to feed for another twelve to eighteen months, and she weaned gradually as a mutual decision between us. I would have been devastated if, having one child, it made a decision to wean as my son did."

I then received two brief accounts from two women who breastfed triplets. Both had remarkably positive experiences, although not without problems. The first is a lyrical piece of writing in which the mother, Elaine Norris, remembers how having triplets tied her into her community in a way that giving birth to her two previous children had not. She then noticed, after writing to me, that this feeling had lasted. She wrote, "I had a special moment a short time ago, with a young mother of a newborn, encouraging her efforts, and realizing that I had a huge emotional investment in her success, even though I hardly knew her."

The second story, from Diane Ingray, includes some practical tips about how to survive with four children under the age of two. In her case she received help from her family, but says that it was having confidence and determination that got her through.

Both stories show how motherhood is not just the effort of an individual, even though the mother is paramount. The idea that any single mother can be left to perform unaided is a sign of a truly uncaring society. Effective parenting is not tenable alone, nor even through the cooperative liaison of two loving parents. It is a web spun by a far-flung constellation of people, working together to weave the cat's cradle that makes a child's life possible.

I

I slung my first two infants around with me everywhere. I nursed them through graduate seminar classes, and church services, and even while teaching undergraduate classes on abstract feminist theories about the sheerly political category of woman.

My triplets were born when my daughter was two and a half and my son was seventeen months. From the agonizing start to the painful end nineteen months later, my experience of breastfeeding them is a memory of deepest commitment, strongest community, and fullest family love.

Hard as it was, I believe I'd have nursed them all till they ran off to college were it not for a nasty mastitis. The peach and silk delirium I experienced during that culminating illness is kind of at odds with the practical, material resources that got me through the challenges of breastfeeding. It put an anomalous light on days after unbearable days of pure determination.

I know two important things: that most mothers of multiples find even the idea of nursing two overwhelming; and without absolute commitment within oneself, supported by the whole community, it would indeed be impossible. I understand further that the intense maternal spaces of birthing and nursing have, for me, been the most liberating genderless spaces of my life.

The resources that carried me through a month of endless pumping while my babies were in the neonatal intensive care unit being tube-fed with my precious little milk, the resources that sustained me through a year of indistinguishable nights and days, that held up against anger at being called an angel in the midst of my most human labor, and that ultimately signify a great challenge as living joy are some of our deepest resources: courage, conviction, understanding, community, and maternity.

I called upon all my physical confidence from a life of outdoors activities, and all my intellectual confidence from an academic career. I had to keep fatigue and soreness in perspective. I had to know exactly what I was doing beyond liberal and conservative ideologies of motherhood. And I absolutely had to have the help of others willing to support my efforts—someone to fold some laundry, someone to take the older children to the park and ice cream stand, someone to bring a smile every Tuesday and cutouts for the kids, and someone to rock a baby to sleep.

Friends became closer, strangers became friends, neighbors walked in without knocking. We have experienced great generosity. It has changed the way I look at people, at possessions, at our home, and at our place in the community. It has changed the way I look at motherhood.

II

I gave birth to my three boys, Christopher, Raymond, and Michael, twenty years ago. I already had one child, Shane, who was twenty-two months when the triplets were born, and whom I'd breastfed for a year. The triplets were nine-and-a-half weeks premature, so I borrowed an electric pump from the hospital, thanks to a kind nurse, who helped me hook up extra tubing so that I could express from both sides at the same time. I would bring the expressed milk into the hospital every day.

I had so much milk I had enough to share with other premature babies in the ward. I think I produced something like three liters a day. Luckily this was before AIDS, so it was an easy, informal thing for mothers to give extra milk to anyone who needed it. I still have milk in my freezer that I can't bring myself to throw out. It's been there forever now, so it can stay.

By the time the boys came home, I was producing too much milk and got mastitis and cold sores. It was ugly! But I continued feeding them for the next two years, gradually weaning them at a mutual pace, so that by eighteen months they were on one feed a day.

When they were babies, I would have one on each breast and a bouncinette in front of me which I'd rock with my foot. Whoever went last got both sides, and would then be first on for the next feed. By the time they were toddlers having the one morning feed, there'd be a huge fight, and they'd pull each other's hair and sometimes get quite violent. But I'd manage to sit them down, and they learned to wait.

I never got far from home. Having four boys under the age of two, even though I had a three-seater stroller, there just weren't many places I could go. We were so tired, we had perhaps five or six hours of broken sleep every twenty-four hours. My husband was a chef on shift work, and he took six weeks' leave so he could help sometimes at night in the first few weeks after they came home.

If one baby stirred, I would sneak out and feed it, then wake the other two so I could do them all together. If two babies stirred, I'd try to feed them both together quietly so the other could sleep. If all three woke, I'd have to wake my husband and he'd come and help.

My mum lived nearby and would come over after work to help tidy up or do some baby-sitting so I could go to the shops. We lived in an apartment, so I sometimes went to her house, where we could spread out a bit. My sister and an uncle also helped, visiting after work, to hold a baby while the others fed, or play with the eldest boy, Shane. They would also greet him first, so he never felt left out. And we bought a video player—Shane was the first person in the house who knew how to use it!

I always felt guilty that I couldn't give the triplets all the attention they needed. Our routine was so rigid, I really couldn't have the closeness that's possible with just the one baby. But breastfeeding meant I could sit down and cuddle and talk with each of them, and make up for lost time.

No one ever needed top-ups with supplement. I had enough milk for their needs, and often they could come back for seconds at the end of a feed. I would also hand-express from one breast while feeding from the other, so as not to waste any milk, and had a huge supply that I'd frozen. I supplied milk to a baby in the hospital with an immune deficiency and to a mother who had adopted and wanted to feed at the breast. She came and took nearly all my frozen milk.

I was determined to breastfeed, but I wouldn't have persevered if it wasn't working. I had so much conflicting advice, I just had to follow my own instincts. My pediatrician told me I wouldn't have enough milk for three, but I knew I did. The first two times the triplets were weighed, they hadn't gained any weight, but they hadn't lost any either, so I had enough confidence to continue. By the third weigh-in they were gaining fast. As for me, I drank at least two to three liters of water a day. And I was very thin!

My advice to other women is that it can be done. But if you can't—as sometimes women with only one child can't—then don't worry. Do whatever's easier for the mother. If she doesn't survive, no one survives.

If the boys were crying I'd just have to calm down and accept it. If they were going to sleep and one cried, I'd shut the door and wait, and usually they'd fall asleep within a few minutes. Mostly they were great babies. It was feed-change-burp and back to bed. When the boys were older, and weren't fighting for their turn, they would often be aware of each other while feeding, and hold hands or touch each other, while Shane played with the third baby and kept him happy. I also had a daughter, after the triplets, and breastfed her as well.

When the triplets were sixteen they used to see Pamela Anderson on TV and say how they wished she was their mum—and how they'd still be on the breast if she was!

Weaning Frankie,
Age Five and a Half

L ike painful breastfeeding, the question of when to wean can incite passionate responses among mothers and those around them. For some, the choice is taken out of their hands when their babies decide to wean themselves at a young age. This can cause sadness, although in some cases it's also welcomed as an opportunity to move on. While breastfeeding manuals will offer advice for overcoming what they call a "breastfeeding strike," most mothers will take their children's cue and let go or accept their rejection without a struggle.

While many standard mothering texts still recommend weaning before the age of one, since it's usually easier, and—so they argue—the nutritional value of breastmilk has diminished, the World Health Organization recommends that no child be fully weaned before the age of two. The anthropologist Kathy Dettwyler has shown that, around the world, anywhere between two-and-a-half and seven years is considered normal, with five to six years (when other primates are weaned) perhaps being the optimum age. But for most Westerners, an older child at the breast is considered an offensive sight, so that mothers who follow the WHO guidelines, or the desires of their children, find they have to restrict their feeding to the home. Many think up secret codes with their children for breasts and breastmilk, and instruct their children not to talk about it, or ask for it, in public.

As one woman wrote in her reply to the questionnaire, "As the babies got to one and two and three years old, it was socially more and more unacceptable and I received lots of adverse comments like 'That's disgusting.' After they were two, I only did it at home." Another woman concurred, although along more conservative lines: "I was also not keen on breastfeeding an older child in public, but happy to in my home. I think that I will continue to feed her morning and night until she is at least one."

Another woman wrote, "I will be sad this time, because I don't expect to have any more children. Having said that, if my daughter doesn't wean herself around her first birthday, as her brother did, I probably won't go past eighteen months of age. I still feel awkward about the idea of feeding a walking, talking toddler."

A mother feeding an older child can feel particularly conspicuous under the current conventions for early weaning in Western countries. Widely publicized cases of state-enforced weaning of older children, such as that of the five-year-old boy in Champaign, Illinois, who was separated from his mother for five months after being "reported" by his babysitter, are even more discouraging.

As Naomi Baumslag and Dia Michels point out in *Milk, Money and Madness*, the decision to wean is "largely influenced by cultural pressures." If breastfeeding can be considered an amalgam of cultural and natural practices, then weaning tends to be almost exclusively the domain of historical and collective decision-making, based on such things as the role of women, the supply of other food and clean water, workplace arrangements, or attitudes toward women's breasts. Some decisions to wean, for example, can be based on the need for large families, where the early return of ovulation is considered important.

Baumslag and Michels write of the Syracuse case in which a mother was accused of abuse, then neglect, for failure to wean her two-year-old. They write: "Only in a culture with no appreciation for breastfeeding could that have taken place. In many parts of the world, a woman would be considered guilty of neglect for weaning a child less than two years old." In Sara Corbett's *New York Times* article on extended feeding in America, she writes, "American women still lag behind many of their foreign counterparts when it comes to willingness to initiate and sustain breast-feeding. . . . In Burkina Faso, the median age of weaning is 25 months; in Peru, it's 20 months; in Nepal, it's 31; while in the United States, most children are weaned at or before 6 months." And in Australia, half the children are weaned at six months. Further cultural differences exist within these countries too. As a study at Brigham Young University recently showed, "Black women [in America] are half as likely as white women to breast-feed their babies."

Among La Leche League and Australian Breastfeeding Association members, it is accepted that the child should initiate weaning, or, if weaning becomes necessary for the mother's health or due to other circumstances, then it should be as gradual as possible. This makes perfect sense for women who are working at home as full-time mothers. But for a woman working outside the home, it's not always feasible, especially if her milk supply is already low. In an ideal world, where mothers received adequate support, and some of the tasks of rearing children were shared more fairly, extended breastfeeding would undoubtedly be more widespread.

Returning to work is a fairly common reason for weaning, or at least the scaling back of feeds, especially where there are no facilities for expressing at work and storing the milk. But there are also plenty of other reasons, as this mother showed in her reply to the questionnaire: "The first one weaned himself at two when I was pregnant and I think the flavor of the milk changed. I weaned the second one at three, because he still had three runny poos a day and I wanted to toilet train him, and I thought the breastmilk was contributing to [this problem]. He still asks me for milk occasionally and I say I don't have any more. He says, 'Yes you do,' and tries to pull up my shirt. I feel fine about it."

For other mothers, a desire to recover some autonomy influences their timing. One mother spoke for many when she wrote, "I am enjoying feeding my baby right now, but I am also looking forward to next year maybe going away for the weekend, or having several glasses of wine . . . or just knowing I can do those things."

While reading the questionnaires, I put together a list of weaning strategies as they appeared. Here are some of them:

"Every time my two-year-old wanted to feed, I offered him Fruit Loops instead. He was completely enthralled."

"I painted spots on my breasts with a felt-tip pen and told my daughter that my breasts were sick."

"I put Band-Aids over my nipples and told my daughter my nipples were broken."

"I put a weak mixture of chili water on my nipples. One taste, and he never came back for more. My husband's mother did the same thing when he was young, but he just told her to go away and wash her breasts!"

"I told my daughter there was no milk left."

"I baked my daughter a Good-Bye Titty cake, around the time of her third birthday, and we held a special weaning party."

"I shifted my daughter from the bed to her cot."

"I put mustard on my nipples. It didn't work."

"I used distraction bordering on bribery, offering a fruit ice block, or putting on a video."

"My husband took our three-year-old son away for a weaning weekend. It didn't work."

And one woman related this story about using rubber beach balls:

It was like being with a junkie for four days. She was twenty months old, and I realized later I should have weaned her when she was one. She was very suckie, and extremely verbal. The first day she screamed and

screamed. But in the midst of her hysteria she blub-
bered out "Balls! Balls!"

She meant those colorful rubber beach balls, of
different sizes, that we used to take with us to the
playground every day. I liked them too. So I gave
them to her and she clutched them, so there was me,
the balls, and her.

Within a second she fell asleep with her head on a
ball. I could then put her into our bed, still clasping
the two balls to her chest.

After the first night she woke up extremely hungry
and just ate and ate. So the second night I laid a plate
of Cruskits beside her head, and for the next two
nights I would lie there listening to her munching.

Perhaps one of the most dramatic weaning strategies of all is
one originating from parts of Russia, where women paint their
breasts black. The child then feels the mother's breasts have
died, or are sick, and is angry with them, but sympathetic toward the mother.

The following story, from Alice Springs in Australia, is
about a woman's now eleven-year-old son who, it seems,
might never relinquish his love of nursing.

Topless bathing had just begun on Bondi Beach in the late 1970s, and I'll never forget my youngest son running down the beach, lunging at the topless glamour girls, shouting, "Feed! Feed!" I decided it was time to wean him.

—Reply to Questionnaire

My son, Frankie, turned eleven in August this year. He was breastfed until he was about five-and-a-half years old—in March of the year he started school—1996. He'd been in family day care for a year from eighteen months, and then in child care and preschool. This extended period of breastfeeding was not due to any earth mother tendencies on my part—I'm probably as far from that type as you can get. I'm loud and bossy, with a low patience threshold.

Nevertheless, I was pretty determined to breastfeed from the start. The spanner in the works from day one was my flat nipples, which my otherwise helpful doctor had unfortunately never inspected at close quarters, and which I just assumed would pop out at the crucial time. As an older mother at thirty-three, and the eldest of seven children myself, I harbored none of the fears about not being able to bathe a baby, or change a nappy, that I had heard other women express. I was far more concerned, rightly as it turned out, about lost sleep and liberty!

Of course the nipples didn't pop out, but were mercilessly

dragged out over several agonizing weeks of what seemed like non-stop feeding, supplementary bottles of soy formula, and hideous late-night and early morning attempts to express milk with a hand pump. (There were no electric-powered ones available in Alice Springs.)

The poor kid couldn't get quite enough of a grip to fill him up, so I'd (foolishly) leave him on for ages, then he'd have a bottle, finally go to sleep, and I'd stagger out to the kitchen and try to express milk! Because he couldn't grip the nipple quite enough, the supply never built up to the maximum, so he'd be hungry again quickly. I worked all this vicious circle business out much later, of course! I had every type of nipple shield—from rubber Mexican hats to the soft silicone variety, enough pawpaw ointment to start my own health food shop, and nipples that were so raw I could barely dry them with cotton wool. If only someone had told me about the little vacuum cups you can wear discreetly under your bra to draw the nipples out gently during pregnancy!

I persevered for so long partly because the thought of carting bottles around in a cooler in the Alice Springs summer held little appeal, and partly because Frankie never gave up trying to get a decent feed for himself. He was a total tit addict from the start, show-ing no sign of rejecting the nipple at any stage. My friend Ann would feed him now and then to give me a break—her son is a day older—and he would, of course, instantly fall into a satisfied sleep.

I spent nine pigheaded weeks trying every suggested approach and dedicating my (many) waking hours to trying to feed a baby, mixing formula, and aiming my nipple at a teacup. Then I decided I couldn't take this lifestyle any longer, and Frankie would have to sur-vive solely on the bottle. I was advised to be firm about it if that was my decision, and this was what I endeavored to do. My resolve lasted a couple of days, during which I sometimes got other people to give

Frankie a bottle, but he'd grab at my shirt looking for a bosom at every opportunity. After forty-eight hours I caved in out of sheer sympathy, and the break turned out to be just what I needed. We were off and running after more than two miserable months of insufficient sleep and rations.

Frankie's addiction was unabated and, less predictably, continued to be so for years to come! He could be away from me for up to two weeks, staying with my mother or sister, and would never forget or reject the breast. I started a law degree in Canberra when he was eighteen months old, and he would go to Melbourne during exam times for a week or two, but absence was never a deterrent. He never complained or asked while he was away, but as soon as I'd see him, he'd insist on picking up where he'd left off.

When he was about three or four, I asked him when he was going to give up the "booby," a term he'd picked up from other kids to replace "mommy drink." He replied, "Never." On another occasion he said, "When I'm as old as Uncle Liam" (who was sixteen at the time). Another reply was, "When I'm old enough to drive a car."

He was completely dedicated and when in Melbourne would cuddle up to my mother's bosoms for comfort at night, although he suggested nothing more, fortunately. My father's joking attempts to tell him he was getting too old for this business were completely ignored. By the time he was around three, it was a twice-daily affair only, and fairly brief at that—five to ten minutes first thing in the morning and again at bedtime.

He was, and remains, an extremely outgoing and independent child, certainly no clinging vine or shy little boy. He spent nights with friends and went off on camping and other trips without me from a very young age with great enthusiasm. Any suggestion of giving up the breast, however, was met with horror.

By about March 1996 I was very close to having had enough. The kid was getting on for six years old, after all. I had earlier decided that when I truly had no more patience for this, that would be it. Frankie was at school, and he certainly wasn't letting on to the rest of the class that he was still on the "booby," so I think he probably knew he was approaching the end of the road. I couldn't see much sign of any milk anyway and hadn't for ages. I was beginning to feel like a human pacifier, or dummy—in more ways than one!

One Sunday night I was on the phone in Canberra to a friend in Darwin. Frankie, who was never keen on bedtime—another reason why the breast was so handy—and who I'd assumed was asleep, got up, sat on my lap, and started unbuttoning my dress, insisting on another drink and complaining loudly when I refused.

That was it. I eventually had to get off the phone and put him back to bed, informing him very firmly that tomorrow would be the last day ever on the booby; he was too old, and it was time to give it away. He wasn't too happy, and there were a few complaints for a week or so, but not what you'd call weeping and wailing. He still asked occasionally for years, however, and even now jokingly does so once in a while! It was his preferred eighth birthday present request—just one more time—but not granted.

I'd been a single parent since he was two and a half, and it's arguable that there was an element of comfort on both sides; however, I suspect it wouldn't have mattered much if his father had still lived with us, such was his determination. Others may find it repugnant, but I think that's a matter of conditioning and common practice more than anything with a logical basis.

Also, because it was so hard to get established, and because he never gave up even when I tried to, I was reluctant to push him off when he obviously liked the comfort of it so much. I've seen lots of kids who eventually lose interest voluntarily, and maybe most would. There are probably some, however, like Frankie, who, given the choice, would hang on a lot longer. I'm not necessarily advocating it, but I don't think it's done either of us any harm.

Children Talking

With barely 3 percent of Western mothers breast-feeding their children beyond the age of two, most children have forgotten about breastfeeding before they can talk. Seeing a naked female breast becomes a rare event in most households; and many children are discouraged from taking a close interest in their mother's breasts once they are weaned.

But as most mothers can attest, children are fascinated by breasts, even if weaned early, and love to touch them and talk about them. A friend of mine has a two-year-old who was weaned at eight months. Each morning he says, "Up! Up!" and points to her shirt. He then presses her nipples with his finger, once each side, saying "Nupples!" And happily wanders off. My own five-year-old son, who has just started school, has recently taken to stroking my breasts to get my attention when he's anxious. It's as if he remembers this was once his hotline for communicating a basic need.

In my questionnaire I asked adults what they remember about their own mothers' breasts. The vast majority could come up with nothing, stating they had no memories, had never seen their mother's breasts, had not been breastfed, and would prefer not to think about it.

Wrote one woman, "It's very taboo and embarrassing to think of [my mother's breasts]. I remember touching them by accident once and being grossed out, finding them soft. I don't remember being held."

Another woman remembers asking her mother, at the age of five, what those things were and being told embarrassedly "bosoms." It was the first time she'd seen them.

One inquisitive child asked her mom if she had two separate breasts or just "one bar" across her chest. "My mother simply answered there were two breasts, but didn't offer any further information."

Those who could provide some associations referred to the smell of perfumes, the feel of clothes, the sound of a soothing voice, or a radio that was playing in the background. Some of those who were breastfed managed matter-of-fact descriptions, such as "Soft and saggy, just like mine." Or, "I've seen my mom's breasts a lot and have never really thought of them as the place I fed from. They're just my mom's breasts."

Two answers were outstandingly loving. They both referred to watching their mother's naked body as she soaked in the bath, a ritual where the children were welcome to sit and chat while their mom relaxed. These are companionable associations, not just the mother as nurturer, but also the mother who has the peace of mind and resources to indulge her own sensual needs. Perhaps not coincidentally, the image is an abundantly liquid one.

The same group of mothers, speaking about their children, offer a more relaxed picture overall than they remember having with their mothers. The questionnaires were full of anecdotes of mothers having their breasts patted unconsciously by appreciative infants, or having their breasts stroked or their hair played with by toddlers. Wrote one mother of her daughter, "While she fed, her hand would snake up into my hair, running the strands through her fingers and twirling my curls. She still likes to twirl my hair when she is in need of comfort."

Others wrote of older children inventing endearing terms for breasts and breastmilk and recalled the pleasure of being able to talk about breastfeeding as their vocabulary grew. One mother of a three-and-a-half-year-old reports, "My daughter discusses my breastfeeding with me often. She loves it and tells me so. She says it's sweet and says she loves my breasts, which she calls 'ninis.' She caresses my breasts and tickles them. She will kiss them if they hurt and jokingly talk to them. I have told her I am happy to nurse her as long as she wants to."

One mother who nursed four children for a total of twelve years wrote of her now grown-up family. "Lily and Jonathan both remember breastfeeding, but the other two don't [since they weaned themselves earlier]. Lily, now twenty-two, says she remembers my breasts being like 'soft pillows' and that she loved the taste of the milk. Jonathan, now sixteen, says he remembers how much he loved breast-feeding, and that he would sometimes 'trick me' by continuing to suckle even though there wasn't any more milk coming. He found that very funny at the time, he said."

The same mother also remembers a conversation with her

son Jonathan when he was almost five, exhibiting his strong sense of family loyalty. She writes, "His weaning was, like Lily's, very gradual. When he was four he started going to nursery school, and I asked him if he thought any of the other kids at his school were breastfeeding. He said, 'Only the happy ones.'"

Another mother remembers with fondness the effect of her daughter being able to speak of her needs. She writes, "My daughter fed until she was almost three. From when she was a toddler she would come up to me and softly stroke my breast to ask for a feed. When she was able to talk she would also say, 'Bes,' (breast) in a soft, breathy voice. It was such an intimate moment, that moment of asking."

Another woman reported getting precise feedback from her children on the condition of her milk. "If I am hot, they comment that my milk is hot!" she writes.

And yet another reports on a mild criticism of her technique, although a bit late to be useful. She writes, "My eleven-year-old remembers lying down and being flipped over to the other side, and didn't like it."

One older sibling of a breastfed baby, who "had gone through much turmoil," was now adapting to her new circumstances by acting out her own farewell. Writes her mother, "While [I was] feeding [the baby] she would come to me and try and cover up my breasts and say, 'Bye bye, delicious milk.'"

The next piece is a collection of short statements selected from questionnaire replies, in which mothers asked their children about breastfeeding and transcribed their answers. In each there is a sense of loving exchange and an honoring of their mothers' breasts that is also very matter-of-fact, uncomplicated by prurience or false modesty.

As Barbara Sichtermann writes in her essay "The Lost Eroticism of the Breasts": "If babies had a language and a script we would have been in possession long ago of a manual of polished love techniques for use between adults and babies. Clinical care and pedagogic concern would be cast onto the rubbish tip of civilization."

⌒⌒

It must be true: babies drink language along with the breastmilk:
Curling up over their tongues while they take siestas—
Mots au lait, verbae cum lacta, palabros con leche.

   —Rosanne Wasserman, "Moon-Milk Sestina"

ℬig boob breasts, right in there. I remember when I was a big kid and I suckled from your breasts. They look like they're big fireballs that have little things that you can put fire on.

They taste like milk. They smell like milk because they have milk inside of them. They feel like they are squishy fireballs.

They would say "Nurse! Nurse!" If they could talk, they could say, "Horse." They mean, "Nurse whenever you want."

   —Girl, age four

It was comforting and relaxing, and I looked forward to it. It was warm.

—Boy, age eight

I don't really remember anything about it, even though I was weaned at a late age. My mother told me about how breast-feeding makes kids smarter. Mum thinks that's why I'm so smart. I don't really think of my mother's breasts as being anything more than part of her body, no different from her arms or legs. I feel a bit awkward thinking about them, to describe the way they look and stuff, like it's nothing I want to give too much thought to. I just think of them as my food source when I was a baby.

—Boy, age seven

The word *addictive* comes to mind.

—Girl, age twelve

I remember how I gave up Mommy's milk. I was three, and I was Batman, and I wanted Mommy's milk. Mommy said to me, "Batman doesn't have Mommy's milk." I was a big boy from then on.

—Boy, age three

They're like big balloons, and there's a knot where the string gets tied on.

—Boy, age two

Can I see? Can I hold it? Can I suck?

—Boy, age six

I remember sitting on my mum's lap and sucking her breast. When my baby brother was born I wanted to try and drink from her boobs as well, but she wouldn't let me. Her breasts are plump and interesting. I relate to them very well. Mum's breasts were my first food source.

—Boy, age twelve

I need it, I need it.

—Boy, age three

Your breasts turn into water and that's why you drink so much water. You have to drink a lot of water to get milk.

I breastfed until I was four and a half. I didn't drink from a bottle. I like the milk, liked it when I was a baby.

My mom's breasts are big and full of tons of milk. They look really thick and have these little doodads on them. They're little and puffy sort of things, small. They smell like breastmilk. They taste like milk. They feel funny, like really really really thick. They're almost way too thick.

They would say to me, "Drink milk." They would say to Mommy, "Drink more water so you can make milk for your kid."

They mean lots of stuff. They're really really neat, and they give me some good milk.

—Girl, age five

They're like googie eggs. They're round and soft, and I can eat them for breakfast.

—Girl, age five

It tastes like Coke! Lemonade in that one, Coke over here.
—Boy, age three and a half

Hello people!
—Boy, age eighteen months, addresssing his mom's breasts

Dreaming

Have you dreamed about breastfeeding? If so, what happened?

I've had dreams about nursing kittens on my breast. I think
that's a symbolic connection to my breasts and my sexuality.

When I was pregnant the first time, I dreamed that my
baby was born with a full set of teeth.

I've had recurrent dreams that I'm breastfeeding a baby
girl, even in my later years.

I dreamed of breastfeeding someone else's baby because it
needed to be fed. I felt ambivalent about the closeness
with someone else's child, but I knew I was doing the
best thing.

Up to Emily being three months old, I used to dream that I
had fallen asleep feeding her. I would dream that she
had either fallen off the bed or was under the bed covers, so I'd go searching for her in my sleep.

I dreamed I was in New Zealand visiting my partner's relatives, who are of Maori descent. In my dream, I am
feeding my Bubs, and he is five years old. Then my
child moves around the room to take turns being fed
from all his aunts and uncles.

I dreamed that milk just spurted up into the air and that I
had no control over it.

I dreamed I had smothered my baby in bed. I woke up in a
sweat, but he was lying, breathing sweetly, beside me.

While I was pregnant with my first child I would dream of
feeding, and couldn't wait to do so.

I dreamed I was breastfeeding twin boys. It was a wonderful feeling and a precognitive dream about me branch-
ing out into two different aspects of my life.

I once dreamed I was breastfeeding kittens. Their little
tongues felt lovely.

I think you need to sleep in order to dream!

I occasionally dream that I am entreating a new mother,
usually someone I know, to breastfeed, but I can never
convince them.

I dreamed about breastfeeding when I was pregnant with
my second and third children and couldn't wait to
breastfeed again.

I dreamed that another woman wanted to breastfeed my
son and I was very upset. I was worried what she may
have had in her system—caffeine, artificial sweeteners,
drugs, or anything else harmful to my baby. Not to
mention that I felt jealous!

I occasionally dream that I'm feeding another baby of my
own. Although I've spent almost three years breastfeeding, and nursed over four thousand times, the experience and pleasure seem way too brief.

I always enjoyed dreaming about feeding kittens and mon-
keys, who were born from me!

I dreamed about being in an earthquake, trapped under
some rubble with my nephews, and having to nurse
them.

I've dreamed more than once this year of breastfeeding,
even though I've not breastfed for nineteen years. I
think it was after caring for my little granddaughter.

I dreamed I was given the choice of breastfeeding a lizard
or a horse. I chose the horse.

For years after my girls were weaned, I continued to have
many dreams about my milk letting down and feeding a
baby. My yearning for breastfeeding eased but never
went away altogether.

White Chocolate

T he last story in the book is about my own breastfeeding experience, and my mother's, and how it played a part in the way our relationship evolved. It includes my mother's account of her experience breastfeeding five children in the 1950s. Although a trained nurse and midwife and married to a doctor, she is impeded every time but once by illness and pregnancy.

Having learned from my mother's story that I was breastfed for only a few weeks, I then looked at the responses of other people to not having been breastfed. How have the several generations of children who were born when breastfeeding was unpopular, many of whom are now parents, made sense of this trend in child rearing?

In answering my survey, most offspring of failed breastfeeders were understanding, even sympathetic toward their mothers, recognizing their limited access to adequate information, and the oversupply of misguided advice. Where a mother tried and failed to breastfeed due to poor care, they were careful to acknowledge this. A New Zealand woman missed out on being breastfed because her mother had severe mastitis with her first child and decided not to attempt breastfeeding again. "She did what was right for her at the time and what was best for me as far as she possibly could," she wrote. "I would not have liked to put her through the excruciating pain of mastitis again, and I appear to have suffered no ill effects."

A significant number of women lament their loss, a sadness that is compounded by empathy for their mothers having missed out too. As one wrote, "In some sense I used [my mother's] feelings to inform my own breastfeeding decisions—her regret did not have to be mine. I also felt her sense of disempowerment very strongly."

Another remembered, "Mom said she really wanted to [nurse me] and would sneak in and breastfeed me when my grandma wasn't home, or at nighttime. I think that is so sad."

One woman told of the way in which her mother's inability to breastfeed was part of a larger picture of loss:

I was put onto a bottle from the very first day. My mother was told that she had no milk for her first child, so was sure it would be the same for the following five children who came along. She found this a great sadness, but was resigned to it. After her sixth child, she had an operation to both wrists for carpel tunnel syndrome. She remembers sitting in a chair holding her tiniest baby in her bandaged arms and trying to feed her a bottle while she had me, only eleven months older than her sixth baby, lying on a cushion at her feet, feeding myself from a bottle. This image fills me with profound sadness, and goes to the heart of my image of motherhood as martyrdom. I picture my mother, depleted from poverty and so much mothering, in pain, and still struggling to feed her two youngest babies. She has built her identity around being an excellent nurturer of small babies, so there is always a touch of sadness and wistfulness when she sees me breastfeed my own children. It's as if she thinks that she can never really lay claim to excellence in mothering because she couldn't breastfeed. Her lips purse up and she tries to be extra generous in her ministrations to me.

Several women speculated on a connection between allergies—asthma, excema, or digestive disorders—and the cows' milk or formula they were given as infants. Yet some of these women still felt empathy for their mother's situation. Wrote one woman, "I am not angry or sad that I wasn't breastfed— more disappointed for my mother's sake that she was never given the support, confidence, and encouragement that she so obviously needed. Both my sister and I suffer from allergies and . . . I know how important breastfeeding is in this regard. I was determined that my two would be given this advantage."

A typical response of those who voiced regret came from a woman who wrote, "I wish I had been fed by [Mom's] breasts; we may have been closer if that had been the case." Another wrote, "I wish someone had nursed me. I am angry for not being nursed and cuddled. And sad."

The angriest response came from a woman in her forties, whose mother chose not to breastfeed her because "She didn't want to lose her figure." With outrage in her voice, she told me how, at three years of age, when her brother was born—and also not breastfed—she watched her mother become ill and "gain a lot of weight." Her mother's efforts to remain slim were not only misguided (since breastfeeding would have more likely contributed to slimness) but futile. Her daughter felt doubly robbed, since her sacrifice had done no good and perhaps contributed to harm.

Another respondent wrote more resignedly, "I frankly have a cynical attitude about my own child rearing, and that I was not breastfed is just another example of its joylessness."

One of the most moving accounts I've read is by the Scottish writer Jackie Kay in her short story "Big Milk," published in *Granta* 63 in 1998. The central character describes watching her lesbian partner breastfeed their child. She is transfixed and jealous, and in love with them both, but unable to enter their charmed circle. As her yearning to be part of this circle becomes more intense, she reminisces about her own mother, who, she writes, "spoon-fed me for two weeks, then left." She begins to imagine herself as a baby being breastfed, "lying across my mother's white breast, my small brown face suffocating in the pure joy of warm, sweet milk." She then gets up in the middle of the night and drives across Great Britain in an effort to find her mother, whom she has never really met, hoping to confront her with her unappeased and reignited longing.

In writing this story, I remembered the time when I was a teenager, and in crisis. I had an intense need for loving guidance, which I could not express, but remember having a longing literally to be held, as though cradled, in an adult's arms. Adolescent angst perhaps doesn't relate to breastfeeding directly, although no study has ever to my knowledge considered such a link. But I came to see this time as a crucible for ongoing difficulties in my family that reached backward to infancy and my mother's problems with breastfeeding and mothering. There were lots of other factors affecting us, and times of real abundance and happiness too. My mother labored constantly, and I have many positive memories that contrast with her tiredness—stirring cauldrons of plum jam, playing Schumann on the piano, and knitting children's sweaters late into the night. But looking back, as most women do on having children of their own, I saw a distinct thread linking inadequate support for families and a wider culture of neglect, to fractured intimacies, and my need for reassurance that my mother was there for me.

In a similar vein, my story also led me to remember the desire I felt as a teenager to be kissed by the man I loved, who was much older, and fundamentally inaccessible. He played an important role as an ill-advised surrogate mentor whom I pursued in a spirit of sexual adventure. But my feelings were also a transference of affection from my older brother, who had recently died. It was a heady brew of love and grief. A time of losing things and having no idea how to replace them, or even begin to measure what exactly had gone missing.

Remembering my lover's aversion to kissing, I was struck, as many people have been before me, by the close relationship between kissing and breastfeeding—these two things, it seems to me now, that had been withheld. I marveled at how it had been too easy to accept the lack of kindness that existed in those early erotic exchanges, where kissing was absent, and how impossible it had been to ques-

236 • Fresh Milk

tion, even register, the lack of warmth that existed at home. I
don't see this as anyone's fault. It was more like being adrift
in a cultural malaise—physically, socially, and emotionally
disconnected.

As Norman Weinstein writes in his poem, "Variations on
a Line of Kenneth Patchen's":

> . . .
> *and if her breasts be lost nothing could*
> *a mind tally*
> *as gain . . .*
> *. . . &*
>
> *if one or both be lost*
>
> *what could replace them in kind*
> *where all kindness in their form*
> *reside?*

As I went on to breastfeed two children of my own in my thirties,
memories and connections emerged in surprising ways. And as I
turned to my mother once again for guidance and support, many of
those early broken threads, those invisible, long-lost filaments,
recovered their warp and weft.

Like swimming, dancing, or making love, breastfeeding must
be learned, and the knowledge of how to do it comfortably
and well (though with many cultural variations) can be lost.

—Nancy Scheper-Hughes

When I was seventeen, and studying for my final exams, I
spent a lot of time at home. I was unhappy, and stressed,
and overshadowed by bogies. My older brother had committed suicide a few years earlier, and I was damaged by this, as well as being
trapped in a teenage depression of my own. I dreaded exams, and
was obsessed with my weight. I used to say I was a failed anorexic, in
a joking way, but I was also worried about being a failed student. I
swung between a desire for thinness, which was partly a desire for
control over a chaotic family drama, as it played itself out through
divorce, and a desire to do well at school. Mostly, the desire for thinness won out.

Around this time I was also having a doomed, sporadic affair
with a doctor, unbeknownst to my parents. He was twelve years older
than me, a sparkling younger colleague of my father. Karl was a
cliché playboy in a sports car, who once collected me outside my high
school, in a brazen Lolita-style dash. But mostly we protected our
secret. I would call him, and then stand outside the cemetery on the
corner of my street, in a haze of nervous agitation, waiting for him to
pick me up and take me to his place, where we'd sometimes have sex,

or go out to dinner. Then he'd drop me home again, or if I'd told my mother I was staying at a friend's place, I'd stay the night. But I never felt at ease with Karl, even when he slept, and would lie awake for hours, my anxiety churning through the night.

In the morning he would drop me off near my house, or I'd walk home across the cemetery, wondering if my brother had a plaque in the cremation garden. If he did, I never found it.

Even though we didn't see each other all that often, I thought about Karl constantly. For some reason he never kissed me, and for years afterward I instructed my boyfriends of the more normal kind that kissing was a sexual platitude, since this is what his aversion, from someone so sophisticated, seemed to suggest. He was also shy about his genitals and never let me see or hold his penis. He smoked constantly, and I used to remark to myself, more bravely sardonic in my head than elsewhere, that he would have made love at arm's length with a cigarette in his mouth if he wasn't so concerned about appearances. Later on, in my thirties, I requested a boyfriend to have sex with me this way, just to see what it was like. He looked comically self-conscious, but I relished the figure he cut—naked, erect, and smoking.

As a teenager, things were not so cheerfully ironic. My most reliable companion was chocolate. As an obsession, it was possibly even bigger than Karl, certainly more dependable and yielding of its pleasures, and almost as much of a secret. Chocolate was my anchor in the stormy inland sea of adolescent mood swings, exam anxiety, romantic obsession, and my fascination with suicide, wanting to know, and sometimes feel, what my brother had been through.

There was a supermarket in the shopping center across the road, which I'd visit every day. I'd put it off as long as possible, which was usually midafternoon. Sometimes I'd walk or ride my bike to a far-away corner store. I was cloaked in shame, and hid my purchases. I always waited till I got home, cocooned with a book or magazine, music in the cassette player, and lying on my bed, or, if the house was empty, on the sofa in the lounge room. I ate mostly large, family-size blocks—Snack, Caramello, Fruit and Nut, Old Gold, Peppermint, Rum and Raisin. Sometimes white chocolate when I needed a change. But most often regular Dairy Milk, which is still a favorite today.

Another memorable thing about this time was my fear of the dark, and I'd sometimes creep in beside my mother late at night, while she slept alone in her double bed, and she didn't seem to mind, too much, my presence there. There was a large tree out back, where my room was, which scraped against the French windows, and possums that would thump like giants lurching across the rafters. But really my fear was a generalized dread, writ large in the darkness.

It must have been on waking in my mother's bed one morning that I first chanced upon her own stash of chocolate. My mother seemed so restrained, and ate such small portions at mealtimes, I was taken by surprise. It was a single four-ounce bar of Cadbury's white chocolate, lying in the top drawer of her bedside cabinet.

For the next few weeks, my routine changed. Instead of visiting the supermarket each afternoon, I would sit on my mother's bed, and take out her chocolate, and eat it. I would then cross the road and purchase an identical replacement block, so my theft would remain secret. I thought each day that I wouldn't do it the next, but inevitably succumbed to temptation. The new chocolate was always there the following day, so my mother never ate it. Perhaps—unthinkable possibility!—she had forgotten all about it.

•

When I began researching this book, I asked my mother whether she breastfed me. Her answer was complicated, so I decided to tape an interview, and this is what she said:

I only satisfactorily fed one of my five babies for any length of time, and that was Penelope. I can't tell you exactly how long, but I do remember her early infancy was very easy and tranquil. The conventional wisdom was that the third baby is the easiest, and in my case it was true.

With my first baby, Anne, I was pregnant again within three months. The breastfeeding so far had gone very well. But on every occasion I became pregnant I would start losing weight, and had a lot of nausea and vomiting. So with the combination of that and my new pregnancy, my milk supply just disappeared.

With Tim, my second baby, there was quite a drama. When he was just two or three weeks old, I developed a severe headache and double vision. Your father, Mick, and his medical colleagues were all in a flap because they were quite sure I had a brain tumor. But then, while Tim was still less than four weeks old, Mick came home with chicken pox. He'd made a house call to a family with chicken pox, and by the time he got there the mother had a ruptured ectopic pregnancy, so there wasn't any hand-washing. Mick was covered with chicken pox, then Anne had a mild attack. Tim was absolutely covered in spots, from one end to the other, and then I had a severe attack too, of the sort when you get it in your throat and absolutely all over. I ran a very high temperature for a few days, and when that cleared, my sight had righted itself, and my milk supply had disappeared.

I had done my midwifery training in 1951, and much of that had been very early care training, because mothers stayed in hospital for anything up to two weeks after a perfectly normal delivery. Assisting a woman to establish breastfeeding before she left hospital was a very important part of my job. We did this with a great deal of conscientiousness. I think I delivered forty babies during my training, and I was working in the ground floor nursery of King Edward Memorial Hospital, where I just fell in love with babies. I topped the state exam for that year, and that included baby care as well as obstetrics.

I was considerably overdue by the time you were delivered, my fourth baby. You were in the breech position throughout my pregnancy, but when you were born you presented a foot and a loop of cord, which was terrifying. You were a somewhat shocked baby. I remember my doctor saying, "Christ!" and then I didn't see you again for another twenty-four hours. After I asked if you were okay, they brought you in to see me, but I don't think I was able to hold you for a couple more days. Eventually I was able to go to the nursery and try to feed you there. All this was complicated by the fact that I had a hacking cough, which I'd had for some time. My milk supply wasn't all that great. So after we went home I would have been supplementing you with a mixture of cows' milk. By the time you were three months old, I was still coughing, and you had a very obvious attack of asthma. The general consensus was that it might be worth trying goats' milk, as there was more and more recognition of the fact that goats' milk was easier for new babies to digest than cows' milk. My main recollection of the time was that you loved it, and thrived on it. The only downside was boiling up the goats' milk, which was horrible smelling, especially if it boiled over.

When Josephine was born, we were living in London, and it was another drama! What else would you expect? I was induced again because I was overdue, and I had edema. But it turned out we'd picked up hepatitis on the boat from Australia. Timothy had gone yellow. And within a day or so of giving birth, I was bright yellow and so was Josephine. I was trying very hard to breastfeed, but I think probably if I went home breastfeeding, it certainly wasn't for more than a week or two.

•

It's impossible to quantify the effects on children of not being adequately breastfed, if at all. My mother and I provide one slender narrative from three postwar generations of mothers and their children who have been imperceptibly pulled apart by the Nietzschean currents of Western science, the corporate greed of formula manufacturers, and—perhaps most important of all—the lack of both practical and emotional support for mothers in our culture. Considering my mother's circumstances, I think we did admirably well. In many ways I am lucky.

My first response to the news of my own story was sadness, but not just for myself, since my mother had been let down by her carers. Although she would say that by the standards of her day she was not neglected, it is hard for me not to notice the absence of family and community support. Not only were we separated for long periods at a crucial time, her own health was allowed to deteriorate while she struggled to care for four children under the age of five. I felt angry on her behalf, and also on my own. More than any one feeling, though, the knowledge that a strongly tactile, intuitive bridge was never forged between us, when it would have been easiest to do so, has helped to explain our relationship, and the dissociated culture out of which it grew.

I don't see the absence of successful breastfeeding as a cause or even a symptom of my relationship with my mother, so much as a metaphor for the challenges we've faced of communicating affection. We had no image bank to draw on, or somatic memory of mutual contentment in each other's physical and emotional presence. I realize now that the absence of the embodiment of love that is breastfeeding simply made it harder to recognize the love that she undeniably extended toward me. As one respondent to my questionnaire explained, speaking of mothering her three children in the 1990s: "Breastfeeding makes me nurturing in a way my culture can't."

My first child was born in 1996, and I breastfed him with fervor, not sure at the time why I was so passionately determined to succeed. I had placenta previa, in which the placenta lies over the cervix, which meant that Brodie had to be delivered by cesarean. Since his birth was taken out of my hands, I focused on perfecting the next contribution my body could make, which was at the breast. He was five weeks premature, so I knew it would be harder for us both, and this added to my wariness of bottles, which might have weakened his desire to suckle. He sweated from the effort of latching on, and would stop every few seconds, his chin trembling as he mustered his forces to continue. He soldiered on in a way that I notice he soldiers on even now, as he learns to read and write. Breastfeeding was his first lesson in the fruits of persevering.

But there was more to it than this physical challenge that consumed us both. I was also fascinated by the continuing symbiosis of our bodies, as mine adapted and his grew, and the unique relationship that breastfeeding encompassed. Breastfeeding demonstrated the real meaning of intimacy, which when used as a verb, *to intimate*, means "to make known." Bottle-feeding reduces the opportunity for a baby "to make known" its needs and personality, substituting a series of measurements calculated by the parent alone—milliliters of formula, parts of water to powder, scales for baby weighing, and four-hour segments of time, if the feeding is based on a schedule. Breastfeeding, especially when offered at the baby's request, requires close attention to opaquely expressed feelings—hunger, tiredness, pain, distress, playfulness, even boredom. It requires the intuitive reading of needs, and the subtle art of registering their fulfillment in mind and body.

The intimacy of breastfeeding also rests on the mutual pursuit of pleasure: the langorous play of tongues and lips, the sweet mingling of warm fluids, soft flesh, and comfort, as need and contentment are held in perfect equipoise. As Freud famously pointed out, "Sucking at his mother's breast has become the prototype of every relation of love." Adrienne Rich put it more simply in her poem "To a Poet," where she writes, "Small mouths, needy, suck you. This is love."

The physical act of putting a newborn's mouth to an adult's nipple is, of course, similar to putting your own mouth to that of your lover's, relinquishing distance and language. If we close our eyes it's because it helps our lips to understand the message being conveyed by our lover's mouth, and to make known our own message in return. Blind and wordless, we use the dialogue of the senses to grapple with each other's wishes. It is a delicate saraband, more intricate and harder to perfect than mere sex, which tolerates more ungainly dance steps. No wonder the lover of my teenage years shied away.

When Brodie was due, my mother flew across the world, from Perth in Western Australia to New York, to help me. She greeted me with happy though jet-lagged weariness, while I was still woozy from morphine and Brodie pitifully weak from his premature eviction. The three of us huddled together in the cramped so-called nursery, really a storeroom of the neonatal intensive care unit at Beth Israel Hospital, figuring out how best to arrange Brodie's splint, used for his drips, and my own intravenous tubing, so that he could reach my nipple.

I had read lots of books on breastfeeding, but none of the diagrams resembled the scene before me now. I had until then been relatively small-breasted, but now I seemed huge. Each of my breasts was larger than Brodie's head, and I couldn't see how his tiny mouth could possibly open wide enough to hold my nipple, let alone any of the surrounding areola, which is what the textbooks assured me was necessary.

It was my mother who took charge, in one swift and gentle gesture. Holding my breast in one hand and Brodie's head in the other, she carefully planted us together.

I brought Brodie home from the hospital two days later, and my mother gave me the present she had brought from Perth. It was a white knitted shawl, which she said she had chosen because my shoulders might get cold during those late-night and early-morning feeds.

Of all the presents a mother might choose, she had lighted upon the one aspect of mothering that I came to be most intrigued by. She didn't know, when she bought it, that breastfeeding would become the subject of a book I would write, or even that I was going to breastfeed at all.

If a gift describes the person who receives it, then my mother knew me well. If it also describes the spirit of the giver, then I was reminded that she had some unfulfilled longings of her own.

Little by little, my mother has given me her white chocolate. It is as pale as the skin on the inside of her arms, and as meltingly smooth.

It is not made of any kind of milk, or sugar. It is not wrapped in foil, or hidden. It is a barely felt connection, the trace of a bond that nearly never was.

And the words in this book are like a vast new shawl, luxuriously cascading from the one she gave me, which I am gladly wrapping around us.

AFTERWORD

❦

We dramatize who we are, every time we eat.

—Margaret Visser

ince I began collecting these stories, the material has continued to seep in. A local newspaper reports that the Federation of Australian Commercial Television has objected to the image of a baby at a breast, part of a breastfeeding promotion campaign, as unsuitable for children's viewing. A divorced mother of three tells me of her fight for custody of her youngest child so that she can wean him at his own pace. A friend tells me of her relief at weaning her five-month-old daughter after struggling to supply her with enough breastmilk. A man calls from interstate on his cell phone to tell me of a Spanish film, *Sleepless in Madrid,* that includes a breastfeeding scene. A girlfriend mentions how much easier it is to feed her second son, now ten days old. Another friend's partner is struggling to feed her newborn.

I sometimes feel like a lightning rod on the subject. It's as if people have lots to say about breastfeeding, but there's a shortage of people to say it to. It's hard to avoid the conclusion that not enough room, time, or resources are set aside in our culture to accommodate and celebrate, or begin to understand, lactation. Despite the official acceptance of breasts being best, breastfeeding is expected to fit into those odd times when it's possible—between sleeps, between jobs, between shopping trips, between whatever other tasks and pressures are crashing in. On the one hand, there is an abundance of milk, and stories about milk, overflowing in the intense weeks and months following childbirth—from dramas of crisis and pain to dreamy love-fests. On the other hand, these milk stories are pushed away, almost before they've been uttered—by stress and sleep, by older children and partners, by images of smiling babies on formula packaging, by everyday routines and outmoded ideas of public decorum.

It seems fair enough that breastfeeding is an incidental part of many people's lives. It can be a transitory, zoned-out time, even for mothers. At times it seems it might become more welcome, if it also became less remarkable. As it stands, the subject of breastfeeding occupies a deeply contested space, and the need for more awareness about lactation has been hampered by the extent to which it has been so thoroughly marginalized, cloistered within the formal exchanges of baby care consultations and the quietly desperate murmurings of mothers' groups.

The stories in this book reach toward a wider, and a wilder, space in which breastfeeding might more freely ebb and flow. They also express a wish to be safe, a basic need that any creature might feel while tending its young. A shopping center mother's room is no such wild place, nor is the average nursing bra. And if we can say these things are safe, then they have come at the price of liberty and joie de vivre. The power of a story is to create a wilderness territory that is also safe—where unorthodox acts, like feeding kittens, making breastmilk ice cream, advertising for a wet nurse, or becoming a breastfeeding father, appear commonplace. These are not feasible in everyone's life, but they contribute to our imaginary possibilities, and to the reservoir of knowledge about the human body as a producer of milk. Left to our own devices we are more productive, and more creative, than we think.

The way forward will continue to present practical challenges. Only by ensuring that women win sovereignty of their bodies, through knowledge, support, resources, and equality, will we be able to breastfeed when and where our children need us to. We need to concern ourselves less with feeding "the right way," and more with the right to feed.

The way forward can also occur on another plane, where we explore the ways in which lactation is a form of embodied self-expression. Like tears, milk is functional; but it also has a lot to say about us. We simply need to replace our fearful, squeamish reverence with openness and curiosity.

If we could expand the boundaries that constrain the body's genius for breastfeeding, by loosening the grip of outdated conventions and attitudes, maybe we could allow it to drift in and out of all our lives, and revel with grace in its pleasures.

RECIPES

◦━━◦

Annuska's Sourdough Bread

This bread takes two or three days to make. Sometimes the dough
doesn't rise. Some people say that if you're a woman, you have a better chance that the dough will rise because women are more "yeasty."
If your dough doesn't rise, try to feed it longer until it does. This is
an adaptation from a recipe in *The Joy of Cooking* (New York: Scrib-
ner, 1997), p. 756. All I did was to replace water with breast milk at
the beginning. I have done it twice, and I got great bread both times.

2 loaves or 4 baguettes

FOR STARTER DOUGH:
½ cup flour
¼ cup warm breast milk

FOR BREAD:
1 cup starter dough
2 cups water
4½ cups flour
1 tablespoon salt
Oil

First, mix ½ cup of flour with ¼ cup of warm breast milk in a clean bowl. Turn it out onto a clean (unfloured) work surface, and knead it until smooth and elastic. Return the dough to the bowl, cover tightly with plastic wrap, and poke some holes in the plastic. Let it stand at room temperature for half a day, approximately.

Repeat this three times, adding ¼ cup of warm water instead of milk, and then give it twenty-four hours to rise. Then do it twice more, or as necessary. The dough should be bubbly and smell a little sour. This is the starter for the bread.

To 1 cup of the starter dough, add 2 cups of water, the flour, and the salt and mix. Adjust the consistency of the dough by adding flour or water. The dough should be sticky to the touch but should not actually stick to your hands. Knead it until smooth and elastic.

Coat the dough with a little oil, and let it rise in a bowl, covered with plastic. It will take less time in a warm place, but a slower, longer rise will make a tastier loaf.

Divide the dough, and shape as you like. Place the loaves on floured wax paper or on oiled cookie sheets. Cover with oiled plastic or a cloth, and let it rise at room temperature until doubled in volume.

Preheat oven to 450°F (220°C). Make some cuts on top of the loaves with a razor blade or a fine knife, as this is essential to help the bread rise in the oven.

Spray the oven with water, wait a minute, and slide in the loaves. Wait a little more and spray the oven walls once more. Bake until browned, 35 to 45 minutes. Turn off the oven and let the loaves stay there for 5 more minutes.

Cool completely before eating.

Gayle's Breast Pump-kin Pie

A Thanksgiving favorite—after all, we have so much to be thankful for as breastfeeding mamas! Share your abundance, your overflowing horns of plenty, with your guests!

> 6 eggs
> 1 can (20 oz.) solid packed pumpkin
> 2 cups brown sugar
> 2 teaspoons granulated sugar
> 1 teaspoon salt
> ½ teaspoon ground cloves
> ½ teaspoon nutmeg
> ½ teaspoon ginger
> ½ teaspoon cinnamon
> 2 cups milk (a combination of evaporated and breast—
>   see below)
> 2 prebaked 9-inch pie shells (store-bought or your
>   favorite recipe)

Beat eggs in a large bowl. Add pumpkin, sugars, salt, and spices. Mix until smooth.

Express breastmilk into measuring cup (up to ¼ cup.) Add enough evaporated milk to make 2 cups of milk total. Gradually stir the milk into the mixture and pour into pie shells. Bake at 450°F (220°C) for 10 minutes; reduce heat to 350°F (180°C) and bake for 40–45 minutes.

Put aluminum foil over edges of pie crust if they look ready to burn. When a knife inserted in the center of the pie comes out clean, it's done.

Let the pies cool on a wire rack before serving. You may want to put a generous mammatocumulus mound of whipped cream or ice cream (breastmilk laced, perhaps?) on top of each slice.

If you think some of your guests will freak out when they discover that breastmilk is a featured ingredient, divide the pie filling into two bowls, and only add breastmilk (from a few squirts up to ⅛ of a cup) to one of the pies. Let your guests know beforehand which is which. (Or see if they can guess!)

Nick's Vanilla Diazepam Ice Cream[1]

Easy to prepare[2] and tasty! Makes one-and-a-half servings.

¾ cup breast milk from an editor at a prominent
   newsweekly[3]
¼ cup organic skim milk
1 teaspoon imitation vanilla extract[4]
1 cup white sugar
1 raw egg[5]

Mix the ingredients in a bowl for a while. Worry about salmonella poisoning. Pour into ice-cream making machine. Let mix until thick (about twenty minutes) while reading Flannery O'Connor stories.[6] Pray for nothing bad to happen. Consider the symbolism.[7] Eat.[8]

---

[1] Before I could meet my friend Jennifer, the editor of a prominent newsweekly, for the handoff of the transfusion bag full of mother's milk, we had an email exchange in which I said that I was both drug-free and allergic to penicillin. Jennifer revealed that she was recovering from a bad infection for which she had been prescribed both diazepam (in the popular Valium brand) and penicillin. It was therefore decided that she would wait a few days for these medications to vacate her system before using the pump to express her bounty on my behalf. For guilty ice cream users and those who might need a little serenity, I therefore suggest you contact a donor who has recently recovered from a bad infection, so that you might reap the benefit of her prescription.

[2] The recipe had better be easy to prepare because if you're like me, you will have many misgivings before embarking on this project. I confess, for example, to some apprehension having to do with the intimacy issues involved. I was about to make ice cream from the extrusions of Jennifer's physique! A day or so passed in which it was clear to me that I was going to throw away the mother's milk in my refrigerator and forget the whole

business. Had it not been for the easy-to-prepare character of this recipe, I'm not sure I would have made it at all.

[3] Our lunch was at a midtown New York expense-account joint. We talked about the new Warren Beatty vehicle (bad!) and about a television writer we both knew. Throughout this light conversation, a MOMA bag sat beneath the table, concealing the two little transfusion bags, one containing the mother's milk with diazepam, one without.

[4] Most vanilla extract has alcohol in it, of course, so I use the fake stuff. If you're ambitious about your ice cream, you might want to try using actual vanilla beans.

[5] I might have worried that I was going to get a dire communicable disease from my kind donor. However, I was more worried about raw eggs and salmonella. What allowed me to go forward, despite my worries, was my past as an abuser of drugs. I took many, many pills in my youth without bothering to ask what was in them or where they came from. I smoked an assortment of unidentified weeds. I am lucky to have had as few problems as I did. I therefore tasted mother's milk with the abandon of youth.

[6] On the night in question, I happened to be composing a paper on O'Connor's stories. Choose a different book if you like.

[7] This is the important part of the recipe. You will not be surprised if I tell you that the results of this adventure were imperfect, at least when compared with fresh Vermont ice cream produced right at the dairy. Mother's milk is not the same stuff, is not rich with the abundancies of fat, and therefore the culinary results of my adventure were imperfect, as I say. It was a half measure in the realm of ice cream. But in spite of this there was something incredibly interesting about the whole experience, about my adventure, and maybe it was because I had never had mother's milk before, maybe it was because I was never held by my own mother at her breast. My mother was performing according to type in 1961 and therefore cannot be held accountable, not entirely. Maybe it was the absence of breastfeeding, maybe it was the narrative of the absence of breastfeeding, whichever, it was also true I was absolutely nauseated by this performance I'm recounting. And yet I had this epiphany on the generosity of the maternal physique, that it can feed others, that it contains all they need for a long time. A child can live a year off the sustenance of his mother, requiring little else but to be held and thus fed. Mothers, I understood for an instant, embody the earthly perfection of generosity. Having produced the swaddled babe in the first instance, having fed it in the second, they are conjoined with the fate of the babe, though feeding the babe might cause cracking of nipples and pain of many kinds. I was nauseated by my performance and I was also moved by it.

[8] I ate. Then I threw out the rest and went back to work.

FURTHER READING

*F*ollowing is a listing of the fiction, poetry, and essays that contributed to my thinking while writing this book. Full publishing details of works quoted in the introductions to each story can also be found here.

"Ancient Egyptian Love Lyric," *The Literature and Philosophy of Ancient Egypt*. Translated by Joseph Kaster.
www.photosaspects.com/snr/poems/anonymous.html.
Angier, Natalie. *Woman: An Intimate Geography*. New York: Anchor, 1999. Quotations in introduction to "I Did It!" come from p. 160.
Ayalah, Daphna, and Isaac J. Weinstock, eds. *Breasts: Women Speak about Their Breasts and Their Lives*. New York: Summit Books, 1979.
Bartlett, Alison. "Breastfeeding in the City: Public Practices and Political Performances." Paper presented to the Association for Research in Mothering Conference, Brisbane, Australia, July 2001.
————. "From Here to Maternity." *Campus Review* (March 7–13, 2001), 11.
————. "Thinking Through Breasts: Writing Maternity." *Feminist Theory*, 1, no. 2 (2000), 173–88.
Baumslag, Naomi, and Dia L. Michels. *Milk, Money and Madness: The Culture and Politics of Breastfeeding*. Connecticut: Bergin and Garvey, 1995: Quotation in introduction to "Weaning Frankie" is from p. 36.
Beral, Valerie, et al. "Hormonal Factors in Breast Cancer." *Lancet,* vol. no. 360 (August 2002), 187–95.
Blum, Linda. *At the Breast: Ideologies of Breastfeeding and Motherhood in the*

Contemporary United States. Boston: Beacon Press, 1999. Quotation by Isadora Duncan in introduction to "Thinking Through Breasts" is from an epigraph to this book.

Bradley-McBeth, Anna E. *I Eat at Mommy's.* Maryland: Big Brain Publishing, 1999.

Brandeis, Gayle. "Mother's Milk: A Dairy Tale." In *The Breast: An Anthology,* edited by S. Thames and M. Gazzaniga. New York: Global City Press, 1995, 210–11.

"Breastfeeding and Induced Lactation in the Ageplay Mommy," www.bloodin-moonlight.com/lgl/lact.html.

Browning, Barbara. "Breastmilk Is Sweet and Salty: A Choreography of Healing." Unpublished paper, 2000. Quotation in introduction to "Thinking Through Breasts" is from p. 1.

Caldwell, Sarah. "The Bloodthirsty Tongue and the Self-Feeding Breast: Homosexual Fallatio Fantasy in the South Indian Ritual Tradition." In *Vishnu on Freud's Desk: A Reader in Psychoanalysis and Hinduism,* edited by T. G Vaidyanathan and Jeffrey J. Kripal. Delhi: Oxford: University Press, 1999: 339–66.

Carter, Pam. *Feminism, Breasts and Breast-Feeding.* New York: St. Martin's Press, 1995.

Christakos, Margaret. "Bits" from the series "Bringing You Up" in *The Moment Coming.* Toronto: ECW Press, 1998, 88.

Churcher, Betty, quoted in Introduction. In conversation with the author, 2001.

Cixous, Helene. "The Laugh of the Medusa," Keith Cohen and Paula Cohen (trans.). *Signs* 1 (4):8 875–93. Cixous quotation on writing in "Thinking Through Breasts" is from "Coming to Writing and Other Essays" in *Cixous,* Deborah Jensen (ed.), Sarah Cornell et al. (trans.). Cambridge, Massachusetts: Harvard University Press, 1991, p. 31.

Cokal, Susann. *Mirabilis: A Novel.* Sydney: Hodder Headline, 2001.

Copjec, Joan. "Vampires, Breastfeeding and Anxiety." In *Read My Desire: Lacan against the Historicists.* Cambridge: MIT Press, 1994, 117–39.

Corbett, Sara. "The Breast Offense." *The New York Times on the Web,* May 6, 2001. www.nytimes.com/2001/05/06/magazine/06NURSING.html Quotation in introduction to "Weaning Frankie" is from this website.

Daniels, Kate. "Disjunction." In *Four Testimonies.* Baton Rouge: Louisiana State University Press, 1998, 82.

Dettwyler, Katherine A. "Beauty and the Breast: The Cultural Context of Breastfeeding in the United States." In *Breastfeeding: Bio-Cultural Perspectives*, edited by Patricia Stuart-Macadam, and Katherine A. Dettwyler. New York: Aldine de Gruyter, 1995, 167–215.

—. "The Hominid Blueprint for the Natural Age of Weaning in Modern Human Populations." In *Breastfeeding: Bio-Cultural Perspectives*, 39–74.

Diamond, Jared. "Father's Milk." *Discover*, 16, no. 2 (1995), 82–87. Quotations in introduction to "That Sense of Yes" are from pp. 83 and 87.

Dibbell, Julian. "Preggo Porn." November 2000/www.artbyte.com.

Dignam, Denise. "Breastfeeding, Intimacy and Reconceptualising the Breast." In *Breastfeeding in New Zealand: Practice, Problems and Policy*, edited by Annette Beasely and Andrew Trlin. New Zealand: Sunmore Press, 1998, 75–94.

Enright, Anne. "Diary: My Milk." *London Review of Books* 22, no.19 (October 5, 2000), 34–35.

Faludi, Susan. *Stiffed: The Betrayal of the American Man*. New York: William Morrow, 1999. Quotation in introduction to "Pumping It" is from p. 543.

Fildes, Valerie. *Wet Nursing: A History from Antiquity to the Present*. Oxford: Basil Blackwell, 1988. Quotation in introduction to "Situations Vacant" is from p. 271.

Forna, Aminatta. *Mother of All Myths: How Society Moulds and Constrains Mothers*. London: HarperCollins, 1998.

Freud, Sigmund. *Three Essays on the Theory of Sexuality*. London: Hogarth Press and the Institute of Psychoanalysis, 1953–1974. Quote in "White Chocolate" is from p. 182. For an excellent account of the connection drawn by Freud between breastfeeding and kissing, see Philips, Adam, "Plotting for Kisses," in *On Kissing, Tickling and Being Bored: Psychoanalytic Essays on the Unexamined Life*. Cambridge: Harvard University Press, 1993, 93–100.

Gallop, Jane. "The Teacher's Breasts" in *Jane Gallop Seminar Papers: Proceedings of the Jane Gallop Seminar and Public Lecture*. Jill Julian Matthews (ed.). Canberra, Australia: Humanities Research Center, 1993, p. 11.

Garrett, Elizabeth. "Mother, Baby, Lover." In *The Rule of Three*. np: Bloodaxe, 1991. Quoted in Greer, Germaine. *The Whole Woman*, 48.

Gibson, James. "Revenge of the Cream Queens." *Juggs* (May 2000), 32–34, 54, 86.

Giles, Fiona. "Fountains of Love and Loveliness: In Praise of the Dripping Wet Breast." *Journal of the Association for Research on Mothering,* 4, no. 1 (Spring/Summer 2002), 7–18.

————. "The Nipple Effect." *Sydney Morning Herald* (May 12, 2001), 1, 10–11.

Golden, Janet, "From Commodity to Gift: Gender, Class and the Meaning of Breast Milk in the Twentieth Century." *The Historian* (Fall 1996), 1–9 (Internet text). Quotation in introduction to "God's Gift" are from pp. 8, 6.

————. *A Social History of Wet Nursing in America: From Breast to Bottle.* Cambridge: Cambridge University Press, 1996.

Gore, Ariel. *The Hip Mama Survival Guide.* New York: Hyperion, 1998. Quotation in introduction to "Letdown" is from p. 78. Quotations in introduction to "Thinking Through Breasts" are from p. 77.

Greer, Germaine. *The Whole Woman.* London: Doubleday, 1999.

Hakansson, Tore. "Sexuality and Lactation." Paper submitted to 7th World Congress of Sexology, New Delhi, 1985.

Hausman, Bernice. *Mother's Milk: Breastfeeding Controversies in Contemporary America.* New York: Routledge, 2003 (in press).

Henderson, L., Kitzineer, J., and Green, J. "Representing Infant Feeding: Content Analysis of British Media Portrayals of Bottle Feeding and Breast Feeding." *British Medical Journal* no. 321 (November 2000), 1196. Quotation from Stuttaford in introduction to "Pressure" is from this article.

Hildebrand, Holly. "Breast Work." In *The Breast: An Anthology,* edited by S. Thames and M. Gazzaniga. New York: Global City Press, 1995, 207–9.

Hite, Shere. "Toward a New Female Sexuality." In *The Hite Report: On Female Sexuality.* London: Pandora, 1976, 527–70.

Huntley, Rebecca. "Sexing the Body: An Exploration of Sex and the Pregnant Body." In *Sexualities* 3, no. 3, (2000), 347–62.

Jacob, Angelica. *Fermentation.* London: Bloomsbury, 1997. Quotation in introduction to "I Did It!" is from pp. 125–26.

Kamani, Ginu. "Younger Wife." In *Junglee Girl.* San Francisco: Aunt Lute Books, 1995, 95–100.

Kay, Jackie. "Big Milk." *Granta* no. 63 (Autumn 1998), 99–110.

Kirkman, Maggie, and Linda Kirkman. *My Sister's Child: A Story of Full Surrogate Motherhood between Two Sisters Using In Vitro Fertilisation.* Ringwood: Penguin, 1988.

Kitzinger, Sheila. *The Year after Childbirth: Enjoying Your Body, Your Relationships, and Yourself in Your Baby's First Year.* New York: Scribners, 1994.

Kunesh, Peter. "Literary Sources of Lactating Godesses." www.darkfiber.com/pz/chapter 5.html. Quotations of scriptural material in introduction to "Lilith's Sad Friend" and "That Sense of Yes" are from this source. Quotation from Adrienne Rich's poem "To a Poet" in "White Chocolate" is also from this source.

Lachapelle, David. *Hotel Lachapelle.* New York: Bulfinch, 1999.

La Leche League International. *The Womanly Art of Breastfeeding.* New York: Plume, 1981.

Leroy, Margaret. *Pleasure: The Truth about Female Sexuality.* London: Harper Collins, 1993.

Lewin, Tamar. "Breast-Feeding: How Old Is Too Old?" *New York Times On the Web,* February 18, 2001, www.nytimes.com/2001/02/18/weekinreview/18LEWI.html.

Llewellyn, Kate. "Breasts." In *The Penguin Book of Australian Women's Poetry,* edited by S. Hampton and K. Llewellyn. Ringwood: Penguin, 1986, 158.

Marin, Lynda. "Mother and Child: The Erotic Bond." In *Mother Journeys: Feminists Write about Mothering,* edited by Maureen T. Reddy, Martha Roth, and Amy Sheldon. Minneapolis: Spinsters Ink, 1994, 9–21.

Mascord, Bronwyn. "Tit Man." *NSW College of Lactation Newsletter* 1, no. 4 (July 1997), 11–13.

Masson, Jeffrey. *The Emperor's Embrace: Reflections on Animal Families and Fatherhood.* New York: Pocket Books, 1999.

Maushart, Susan. *The Mask of Motherhood: How Mothering Changes Everything and Why We Pretend It Doesn't.* Sydney: Random House, 1997. Quotation in introduction to "Pressure" is from pp. 202–203. Epigraph to "Pressure" is from p. 204. Quotation in the epigraph to "Hell Ride" is from p. 212.

McBride, James, ed. *M.I.L.K.: A Celebration of Humanity.* New South Wales: Allyons, 2001.

McConville, Brigid. *Mixed Messages: Our Breasts in Our Lives.* Harmondsworth, England: Penguin, 1994.

Minchin, Maureen. *Breastfeeding Matters: What We Need to Know about Infant Feeding.* Melbourne: Alma Publications, 1985.

Moorhouse, Frank. "Late Families, Former Mistresses and Breast-feeding, and the Slowing of the Fast Crowd." In *Late Shows.* Sydney: Pan Macmillan,

1990, 15–20. Quotation in introduction to "Thinking Through Breasts" is from p. 18.

Nagourney, Eric. "Patterns: Breastfeeding Found to Vary by Race." *New York Times on the Web*, August 7, 2001. www.nytimes.com/2001/08/07/health/children/07milk.html. Quotation in introduction to "Weaning Frankie" is from this article.

O'Brien, Pauline. *Discovering Childbirth and the Joy of Breastfeeding*. Sydney: Angus and Robertson, 1979.

Olds, Sharon. "The New Mother." In *The Dead and the Living*. New York: Knopf, 1984, 53.

Oxenhandler, Noelle. *The Eros of Parenthood: Explorations in Light and Dark*. New York: St. Martin's Press, 2001.

———. "Spilled Milk." December 2000. www.nerve.com/dipatches/Oxenhandler/spilledmilk//main.asp. Quotation in introduction to "Tran" is from this source.

Parks, Patrick. "The Cheesemaker's Tale." In *The Breast: An Anthology*, edited by S. Thames and M. Gazzaniga. New York: Global City Press, 1995, 26–30.

Phillips-Thoryn, Claire. "The Sacred Breast: Early Christian Experiences of the Physical and the Divine. The Breast in Medieval and Renaissance Christianity." December 17, 1999. www.sccs.swarthmore.edu/users/02/clairept/sacredbreast.html. Quotations in introduction to "I Did It!" are from this source as is the epigraph to "Lilith's Sad Friend."

Randolph, Dawn. "Milk." www.cleansheets.com/archive/archfiction/randolph-_12.8.99.html.

Raphael, Dana. *The Tender Gift: Breastfeeding*. Englewood Cliffs, N.J.: Prentice-Hall, 1973.

Raphael, Dana, and Flora Davis, *Only Mothers Know: Patterns of Infant Feeding in Traditional Cultures*. Connecticut: Greenwood Press, 1985. Quotation in introduction to "Pressure" is from p. 116.

Rich, Adrienne. *Of Woman Born*. New York: W.W. Norton, 1986. Quotation in introduction to "Tran" is quoted in Natalie Angier, *Woman: An Intimate Geography*, 170.

Rukeyser, Muriel. "Night Feeding." In *Mother Songs: Poems for, by and about Mothers*, edited by Sandra M. Gilbert, Susan Gubar and Diana O'Hehir.

New York: W.W. Norton, 1995, 65–66. Quotation in introduction to "I Did It!" is from this poem.

————. "Pouring Milk Away." In *The Collected Poems of Muriel Rukeyser.* New York: McGraw-Hill, 1978, 414.

Salmon, Marylynn. "The Cultural Significance of Breastfeeding and Infant Care in Early Modern England and America." *Journal of Social History* 28, no. 2 (Winter 1994), 247–67. Quotations in introduction to "I Did It!" are from pp. 247, 249.

Schappell, Elissa. "Here Is Comfort, Take It." In *Use Me.* New York: William Morrow, 2000, 285–320.

Scheper-Hughes, Nancy. *Death Without Weeping: The Violence of Everyday Life in Brazil.* Berkeley: University of California Press, 1992. Epigraph to "White Chocolate" is from p. 326.

Schmied, Virginia. "Connection and Pleasure, Disruption and Distress: Women's Experience of Breastfeeding." *Journal of Human Lactation* 15, no. 4 (1999), 325–33.

Shanley, Laura. "Milkmen: Fathers Who Breastfeed." http://ucbirth.com/milkmen.htm. Quotations in introduction to "That Sense of Yes" are from this website. Quotations from email correspondence by permission.

Sichtermann, Barbara. "The Lost Eroticism of the Breasts." In *Femininity: The Politics of the Personal,* edited by H. Gyer-Ryan. Translated by J. Whitlam. Cambridge: Polity, 1986, 55–68. Quotations in introduction to "That Sense of Yes" and "Children Talking" are from p. 67.

Smith, Julie. "Human Milk Supply in Australia." *Food Policy* no. 24 (1999), 71–91.

Spadola, Meema. *Breasts: Our Most Public Private Parts.* Berkeley: Wildcat Canyon Press, 1998.

Sparkes, Alison. "Spare a Drop?" www.ivillage.co.uk/pregnancyandbaby/baby/feedbaby.

Stearns, Cindy A. "Breastfeeding and the Good Maternal Body." *Gender and Society* 13, no. 3 (June 1999), 308–25.

Steinbeck, John. *The Grapes of Wrath.* London: William Heinemann, 1941, 552–53.

Steinem, Gloria. "If Men Could Menstruate." In *Outrageous Acts and Everyday Rebellions.* New York: Flamingo, 1983, 337–40. Quotation in introduction to "That Sense of Yes" is from p. 338.

Steingraber, Sandra. *Having Faith: An Ecologist's Journey to Motherhood.* New York: Perseus, 2001. Quotation in introduction to "Adopting Elizabeth" is from LACNET Discussion Group Posting, June 10, 2001, with permission.

Svitil, Kathy A. "Prenatal Palates." *Discover* 21, no. 11 (November 2000). (Internet text) Julie Mennella quotation in introduction to "God's Gift" is from p. 1.

Tagge, Mary E. "Wet Nursing 2001: Old Practice, New Dilemmas?" *Journal of Human Lactation* 17, no. 2 (2001), 140–141. Epigraph to "The Other Woman" is from p. 140.

Thames, Susan, and Marin Gazzaniga, eds. *The Breast: An Anthology.* New York: Global City Press, 1995.

Thomas, D. M. *The White Hotel.* New York: Viking, 1981, 22–23.

Traina, Cristina. "Maternal Experience and the Boundaries of Christian Sexual Ethics." *Signs: Journal of Women in Culture and Society* 25, no. 2 (2000), 369–405.

Updike, John. *Couples.* New York: Knopf, 1979, 311–314.

Van Esterik, Penny. "Breastfeeding and Feminism." *International Journal of Gynecology and Obstetrics* 47 Suppl. (1994), 541–51.

Visser, Margaret. "The Comfort Zone," ABC National Radio (Sept. 7, 2001). Quoted in the epigraph to the Afterword.

Warner, Marina. "The Milk of Paradise." In *Alone of All Her Sex: The Myth and Cult of the Virgin Mary.* London: Vintage, 2000, pp.192–205.

Wasserman, Rosanne. "Moon-Sestina," in Thames and Gazzaniga (eds.), *The Breast.* Op.cit. pp. 84–85. Quoted in epigraph to "Children Talking."

Weisskopf, Susan. "Maternal Sexuality and Asexual Motherhood." Review Essay, *Signs: Journal of Women in Culture and Society* 5, no. 4 (1980), 766–82.

Wilson-Clay, Barbara, and Kay Hoover. *The Breastfeeding Atlas.* Austin, Tex.: LactNews Press, 1999.

Winton, Tim. *The Riders.* Sydney: Pan Macmillan, 1994, 190.

Yalom, Marilyn. *A History of the Breast.* New York: Ballantine, 1997. Epigraph to "The Secret Life of Nipples" is from p. 16; quotation in introduction to "The Other Woman" is from p. 45.

Young, Iris Marion. "Breasted Experience: The Look and the Feeling." In *The Politics of Women's Bodies: Sexuality, Appearance, and Behaviour,* edited by R. Weitz. New York: Oxford University Press, 1998, 189–209.

Zepeda, Gwen. "Breastfeeding." www.hipmama.com. Quotation in "Thinking Through Breasts" is from this source.

CREDITS

Many of the stories in this book were told to me anonymously. Some stories were told to me by single voices, others I put together from several voices, and from replies to the questionnaire. The following credits go to those who contributed written pieces that were adapted for this book, and to those interviewees who wish to be named.

"Mammatocumulus," © Gayle Brandeis.

"Letdown," © Belinda Luscombe.

"Thinking Through Breasts," © Alison Bartlett, adapted from "Thinking Through Breasts: Writing Maternity." *Feminist Theory* 1, no. 2, (2000), 173–88.

"Bits," © Margaret Christakos, from the series "Bringing You Up." In *The Moment Coming*. Toronto: ECW Press, 1998, p. 88. Reprinted with the permission of the author.

"Breasts" by Kate Llewellyn. Reprinted by arrangement with Kate Llewellyn. © care of Curtis Brown (Aust.) Pty. Ltd.

"Pumping It" as told by Ed Deroo.

"God's Gift" as told by Shelley Abbott.

"Situations Vacant" as told by Beth Taylor.

"The Other Woman" as told by Pam Sutton.

"Pressure" as told by Liz Banks.

"Feeding Triplets" as told by Elaine Norris and Diane Ingray.

ACKNOWLEDGMENTS

My heartfelt thanks go to the hundreds of women and men who replied to my questionnaire. Your answers have been invaluable in providing background information about the place and meaning of breastfeeding in our world, and in providing insightful, startling, funny, and touching comments for inclusion in this book.

I also wish to thank the many people who told me their stories in interviews, which were then used as background, or for chapters in their own right.

I am grateful to all the people who generously shared both scholarly and personal information with me: academics, breastfeeding advocates, lactation consultants, midwives, journalists, friends, and interested individuals with a story to tell.

Specifically, I wish to thank the following people who gave of their time and resources: Debra Adelaide, Kathy Albury, Stuart Allison, Jonathan Ames, Rita Armstrong, Alison Bartlett, Bruce Bauman, Elyane Brightlight, Barbara Browning, Patrick Bucklew, Erica Chapuis, Margaret Christakos, Christen Clifford, Vanessa Coates, Felicity Copeland, Kate Daniels, Susan D'Arcy, Shaun Davies, Maryanne Dever, Julian Dibbell, Denise Dignam, Janice Eidus, Sarah Emery, Ros Escott, Keren Epstein-Gilboa, Michele Field, Grace Fimbel, Rod Fontana, Leila Forde, Faulkner Fox, Courtney Gibson, Anne Giles,

Cassandra Graham, Karleen Gribble, Rachel Hall, Dian Hanson, Bernice Hausman, Joy Heads, Adele Horin, Rebecca Huntley, Cathy Jenna, Ginu Kamani, Yael Kanarek, Rachel Knepfer, Maggie and Linda Kirkman, Mary Lantry, John Lee, Bill Levy, Catharine Lumby, Margot Mann, Louise Marshall, Bronwyn Mascord, Jeffrey Masson, Dia L. Michels, Maureen Minchin, Jeanne Mitchell, Pauline O'Brien, Clarissa Patterson, Glen Ralph, Rochelle Ratner, Bronwyn Rennex, Tim Rowse, Laura Shanley, Amruta Slee, Kym Smythe, Janyce Stefan-Cole, Joel Stein, Joey Strange, Jenny Todd, Penny Van Esterik, Silvia Velez, Judith Whelan, and Barbara Wilson-Clay. Also to my erudite wine-tasting friend. And to the late Colin Hood, who helped me at so many levels, with his fine intelligence and loving support.

For reading draft chapters from the manuscript, I am sincerely grateful to: Richard Andrews, Bruce Bauman, Lily Brett, Phil Davis, Janice Eidus, Josephine Giles, Joy Heads, Lisa Hill, Colin Hood, Ginu Kamani, Belinda Luscombe, Rick Moody, and Fiona Place.

For looking after me on my travels: Bruce Bauman, Lily Brett, Jeremy Edmiston, Douglas Gauthier, Michelle de Kretser, Belinda Luscombe, Maureen Minchin, David Rankin, Barbara Wilson-Clay and Suzan Woodruff.

To my agents, Elaine Markson in New York, for her encouragement, suggestions, and support; and to Fiona Inglis in Sydney, for her generous advice. To my publishers and editors: David Rosenthal, Marysue Rucci, and Tara Parsons in New York; and Sophie Cunningham and Emily O'Connell in Melbourne and Sydney, for keeping the faith, and sharing in my wonder about this little-understood subject.

To Bill and Louise Luscombe, for the generous use of their beach house in Killcare, which enabled me to see the book whole, and begin to write.

To Paula West and all the staff at Kangas House Day Care Center, for looking after my children while I worked.

To my husband, Richard Andrews, and my two boys, Brodie and Hugo, for accommodating my work, and respecting my need for the closed study door. And not least of all for helping to keep me in touch with my own breasts.

I wish also to pay homage to the work of Shere Hite and Eve Ensler. In the words of Michael Tausig, "It is always a way of representing the world in the roundabout 'speech' of the collage of things. . . . It is a mode of perception that catches on the debris of history. . . ."

And finally I wish to thank my mother, Patricia Giles, for telling me her story with such honesty, passing on information as it came her way, and accepting her intense and uncompromising third daughter. This book was conceived in the spirit of your own work: to promote loving kindness, and strive for change.

ABOUT THE AUTHOR

FIONA GILES is an Australian scholar, writer, and feminist. A graduate of Oxford University, she lives in Sydney with her partner and two sons.